Praise for *Motherf*cked*

"Men often tell me that their dysfunctional relationship with their mother left them ill-equipped for adult relationships with women, and we spend months or years trying to undo the damage. With a combination of research, expert guidance, the author's personal experience, and the most practical, specific steps I've ever seen in a self-help book, *Motherf*cked* is now my go-to recommendation for anyone who's experienced this dynamic, as well as the therapists, coaches, and loved ones who walk with them."

—Ryan Howes, PhD, ABPP, clinical psychologist

"Imagine your bestie just happens to be a psychologist and she's sitting you down for one of those casual yet deeply soul-healing chats, the kind that leaves you feeling fully seen and so much lighter. THAT is the gift Ashley gives the world through *Motherf*cked*. This book breathes validation and hope into an integral yet often impossibly heavy topic, and I am a better woman and daughter for reading it."

—Kelsey Wells, mental health–focused fitness trainer,
women's empowerment advocate, motivational
speaker, and creator of Redefine Fitness

"Ashley Oerman blends soul, storytelling, and expert-backed straight talk to help you untangle from manipulation, guilt, and emotional chaos—and finally come home to yourself. This is a book about freedom and about living your highest, most authentic human experience. With fierce compassion, humor, and hard-won wisdom, she shows you how to set boundaries without guilt, stop over-functioning to earn love, and live as the person you really are. *Motherf*cked* is equal parts healing and healthy rebellion—a guide for anyone ready to stop repeating old patterns and start choosing themselves."

—Susie Moore, host of the top-rated *Let It Be Easy* podcast

"The ultimate traveller's guide to navigating your relationship with your mom: vulnerable, thoughtful, practical, and hugely necessary."

—Jemma Sbeg, host of the *The Psychology of Your 20s* podcast

Motherf*cked

Motherf*cked

How to Stop Your Mother's Toxic Drama from Ruining Your Life

Ashley Oerman

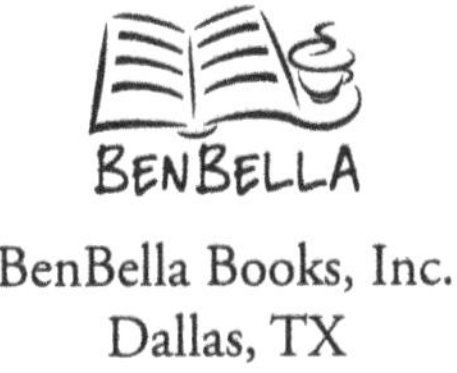

BenBella Books, Inc.
Dallas, TX

BenBella Books, Inc.
8080 N. Central Expressway
Suite 1700
Dallas, TX 75206
benbellabooks.com
Send feedback to feedback@benbellabooks.com

BenBella is a federally registered trademark.

Printed in the United States of America
10 9 8 7 6 5 4 3 2 1

Library of Congress Control Number: 2025047759
ISBN 9781637748619 (trade paperback)
ISBN 9781637748626 (electronic)

Editing by Leah Wilson and Victoria Carmody
Copyediting by James Fraleigh
Proofreading by Cheryl Beacham and Ashley Casteel
Text design and composition by PerfecType, Nashville, TN
Cover design by Emily Weigel
Cover image courtesy of Andrew W. Miller Collection
Printed by Lake Book Manufacturing

CONTENTS

FOREWORD

Minaa B., MSW, LMSW

When Ashley reached out, asking me to share my expert opinion on parent–child relationships for her book, I was thrilled to contribute. With insights, advice, and practical tips from licensed mental health pros like me, as well as research and some of her own experiences, *Motherf*cked* is essential for adult children healing from relationships with their moms.

I have been a therapist for nearly ten years, primarily working with adult clients managing anxiety, depression, and complex PTSD. A lot of my practice is focused on helping people function in a healthy way within their families and heal through community care—a practice I discuss more in my book *Owning Our Struggles*. I also created The Siblinghood Theory, which explains how sibling bonds—biological or chosen—shape people in adulthood, and I spent several years working in Early Head Start in New York City, supporting children and equipping their parents with tools to foster secure attachment relationships.

Whether I am working with a client who's in conflict with their sibling, a child struggling to regulate their emotions, or someone managing trauma, I am constantly examining the relationships people have with their parents—oftentimes, their mothers. What I've come to find is that, no matter a person's age, the desire to be loved and cared for by our mothers never fades, and a lot of damage occurs when that relationship is dysfunctional, unsafe, or unhealthy.

This book isn't a takedown of mothers. As Ashley acknowledges throughout *Motherf*cked*, moms are humans just like the rest of us. That means they, like anyone, can lack the emotional maturity necessary to foster healthy relationships. They might also face obstacles, like socioeconomic struggles and mental health conditions, that make being an excellent parent nearly impossible.

However, the book provides a much-needed check on the mother–child relationship that society often puts on a pedestal. The reality of having a tough dynamic with your mother is one so many have experienced but aren't permitted to call out or, if they do, they're demonized for doing so. This book is the permission slip many people need to finally start addressing the painful parts of their relationships with their moms. It serves as validation for those who have endured the loneliness that comes with this specific kind of struggle.

I've found that adult children don't expect their mothers to be perfect, and they don't deny their moms' lived experiences. Instead, they're asking for emotional attentiveness, affection, care, and curiosity. Adult children want their mothers to acknowledge the impact of their parenting choices, even when those choices were well-intentioned.

Aided by thorough research and lived experience, Ashley unpacks why our feelings about our moms can feel so complicated. She breaks down critical concepts, like attachment styles, emotional immaturity, and boundaries, in ways that will make you feel seen and understood. Finally, and most importantly, she points readers toward a path forward, empowering you to accept this relationship for what it is and make choices based on that truth. Whether your mother is abusive or just hard to get along with, as Ashley mentions, we're all a little motherfucked. This book serves as a guide to get you through.

INTRODUCTION
To Be Honest, We're All a Little *Motherf*cked*

It was the last night of my bachelorette party, and I emerged from a mild blackout, sobbing on a couch surrounded by my friends. I was trauma dumping all over them. Up until this point, the vibes were vibing. And then, apropos of nothing, I melted down in front of a captive audience. This is what the pros call leaking, or letting your emotions seep out when your willpower to shove them down fails (see: you drink tequila straight from the bottle). Though, honestly, this was more like emotional projectile vomiting than some casual leakage. I don't remember exactly what I said, but the subject matter of this wasted, 1 AM lecture? My very complicated, low-key-painful feelings about my mom.

About a year before that purge, I started therapy for social anxiety. At the time, I was an editor at *Cosmopolitan*, and in every monthly editorial pitch meeting, I'd struggle. Those meetings were a big deal. They're where all the editors pitched their ideas for what their sections of the magazine would look like in the next issue. Each time it was my turn, I couldn't read the words on my pitch memos, and it became hard to breathe. Just writing up my ideas for the meeting and printing them out made the heart rate monitor on my Apple Watch go, "Hey, you good?" I t'was not.

It took a while for my therapist and me to figure it out, but my debilitating anxiety was just a souvenir from the mothership. More specifically, I didn't want to be seen in the same way I saw my mom. Awesome. I felt like an embarrassing cliché. Blaming your mom? In therapy? Groundbreaking.

Here's what took me six years to figure out: Emotional manipulation is often part of my mom's maternal love language (consciously or not). From her parentifying me (as the therapists say) as soon as I was old enough to be more than an accessory, to having little interest in me as an adult (much less in my feelings about all that), I do have some notes for Foxy. (Foxy is a nickname for my mother that I use to minimize the emotional impact of her behavior—that's marketing magic, baby. I'll be referring to her this way throughout our journey together. Enjoy!)

It took many uncomfortable phone calls and a couple of emails to deliver this critique straight to its source, and my mom's reception was anticlimactic. Despite my detailed recaps of how she'd hurt my feelings and offering turn-by-turn directions to a better relationship, Foxy still said she didn't understand the problem. "That's in the past. Let's move on," would be her *Real Housewives* tagline.

If you can relate, even a little bit, I see you; I *am* you. As much as it sucks to be a casualty of your mom's limited emotional capacity and/or self-awareness, there's a reason the matriarchy can make us feel shitty: We're born to stan our caregivers from Day One because our survival and development depends on them.

For people who've had happy, healthy, secure mom–child relationships since birth, that born fandom is just a fun fact. For the rest of us, it's the reason we're googling "What is my attachment style?" and "Signs of a narcissist."

We're wired to depend on our caregivers for unconditional love, support, and self-esteem. That's different from other relationships in our lives. So, when our moms aren't able or willing to bring their best selves to the mom game, they set us up to fail.

Still, I have to admit that the tyranny of the human reproductive system (plus the cultural and societal kinds of tyranny) has exerted undue pressure upon moms. And, as we know, not all moms have a stacked roster of positive coping mechanisms, emotional intimacy skills, or mental health pros to assist them through the drop-kick that is becoming a parent.

These days it's common to throw out a "Hurt people hurt people" to explain away messed-up behavior, but that concept does track when it comes to parents. In her book *Adult Children of Emotionally Immature Parents: How to Heal from Distant, Rejecting, or Self-Involved Parents*, clinical psychologist Lindsay C. Gibson, PsyD, explains how childhood pain and trauma in our parents' lives can stunt their emotional growth. Parents who lack basic skills like empathy and accountability and have low self-esteem as adults were often shamed, punished, or judged by *their* caregivers for having feelings as children. According to Dr. Gibson's clinical experience, when people aren't allowed to express or feel emotions, they can come up with really creative, messy ways to avoid feeling things in general.

Issues can also arise if your mom experienced trauma or other extremely challenging circumstances after childhood, including chronic illness, a demanding job (or jobs), precarious economic status, ongoing mental health struggles, or just blissful ignorance of early-childhood development. All of that (and more) can inhibit even the most well-intentioned caregivers.

The result: Some parents can't deal with their own emotions or yours. Ultimately, that can leave us feeling insecure with our moms, in other relationships (platonic or not-that-platonic), and within ourselves.

And yet! Messy relationships with our moms don't have to leave us forever motherfucked.

This book is a primer on problematic relationships with our moms from the perspective of a mental health journalist and editor who's read all of the self-help books, interviewed the most reliable sources, and done the work to recover. It explains why the bond with our moms is such a big deal and where those relationships go wrong. It also digs into the repercussions of these painful dynamics, with insights from mental health professionals who see this situation all the time.

We'll also take a tour through the ways in which our moms' unfortunate behavior in our childhoods can mess with us in adulthood. From actual abuse to the gray area of emotional manipulation, we'll address it all—even that seemingly benign, "I'm just worried about your health" brand of body shaming specific to so many moms—and break down its toll.

But we're not just learning here. We're doing. You'll get specific advice and exercises for healing (and, of course, an explanation as to what the fuck that word even means). We'll also cover strategies for drama management: how to accept your mom as they are now, grieve what they'll never be, address the issues in your relationship, and communicate your boundaries.

You'll also explore whether estrangement—going low- or no-contact—may be helpful for your situation and how to approach that. Last, and most important, you'll hear from other people who've been motherfucked about how they're doing now.

Persistent and thorough mental health reporting during my nine-to-five—and therapy on my lunch break—have helped me start feeling like myself, maybe for the first time ever. It also enabled me to get here, writing this book for you—and also for me.

My progress was so damn slow, though. I mean, maybe that's just how this works—but still. First, I had to accept that my issues with Foxy are real, grieve what that relationship took from me (definitely not in that order), and evolve out of feeling gross and different because of it. Then I had to break patterns I'd kept up out of obligation, set boundaries, figure out how to tell my mom the way she treats me isn't cool, set more boundaries, and deal with people who didn't understand the problem. (I'm tired. Thanks for asking.)

I'm also convinced that if unhealthy relationships with moms were normalized in the first place, I would've arrived here so much faster. Yep, therapy and research helped me sort through the trash pile of self-doubt, anxiety, and just a touch of depression, but the thing that made me feel most OK was talking to nonprofessionals about it. Most of the friends I opened up to (and a few strangers who innocently triggered my mom-shaped emotional baggage) can relate. Turns out, a lot of us have residual mom energy keeping us from evolving into our fullest, hottest, most ~healed~ selves. Still, I'm pretty sure almost none of them would've brought up their issues if I hadn't gone first.

That's why I wrote *Motherf*cked*: to bust through the fuckery of shame associated with having a weird (at best) relationship with your mom and healing from it.

I promise this is not a takedown of momkind. Moms are people—and people are really flawed. However, when those flaws make us, the spawn, feel unloved, the result is more anxious, sad, stressed, depressed humans, which sucks.

That shit stops here—with you. By the time we're through, you'll feel seen, empowered to move forward, and less likely to impulsively drunk-cry about this ridiculously common strain of emotional trauma—or at least be less embarrassed about it when you do. After all, it's *not* just you, it *is* a big deal, and you *can* start to feel better right now.

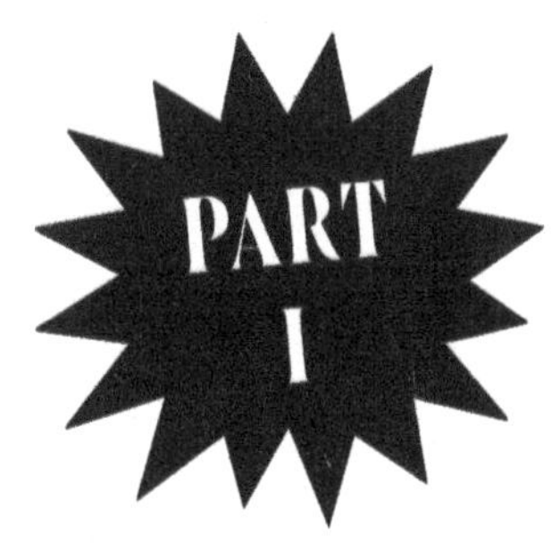

*Why We're Motherf*cked*

CHAPTER 1
Our Moms Matter

A couple of quick notes before we dive in. After wrapping up my research, I believe much of the advice and many of the insights in this book could be applied to a dysfunctional relationship with any primary caregiver, whether or not they're your mom. But because moms occupy a specific place in our cultural imagination, as I'll detail later, I set out to write about what happens when the role of mom is filled by someone whose behavior seems at odds with the ideal, feel-good relationship we're often promised.

Also: While I sometimes refer to your mom as she, her, *or the person who gave you life, please know that I'm still talking about your primary caregiver, whatever form they take. Unfortunately, the damage doesn't discriminate.*

And, last, I just want to throw this out there: I'm a middle-class white woman from the Midwest writing about her relationship with her mom. Despite the specificity of my own experiences, I'm hopeful that anyone who has a tough relationship with their mom can relate to most of what's in here, regardless of your identity or your caregiver's.

I think we can all agree that the people raising the future of humanity are busy, important, and truly underappreciated, underpaid, and underrepresented. Most moms put their bodies, brains, and bank accounts on the line to sustain life—and, oftentimes, to giveth life in the first place.

And if you believe your Instagram feed on Mother's Day and back-to-school ads, you'd assume every mom is happy to fuck around with everything I just listed to find out how amazing their kids will be.

They brought us into existence! They put us on their unlimited plan for unconditional emotional support! They prioritized our every need! They're our biggest cheerleaders! Our number one fans! They know us better than anyone else! They're! Our! Best! Friends!

Except when they don't and they're not. It's confusing to hold these two truths at once. Yes, being a parent, especially in the US (see: lack of affordable childcare, healthcare, etc.), is exhausting unpaid labor (of love—usually). But painting every mom as the patron saint of selflessness and care isn't accurate either.

Not all moms are out here dropping love notes in lunchboxes, doling out couch snuggles, or embracing their kids' weirdo phases. Some moms might not even realize their kids want or need anything like that. Others may think that's actually bad parenting.

What I'm trying to say is that while the intensity of being a mother is a given, healthy, beautiful, captionable relationships for the kids involved isn't. Like a Doordashed Taco Bell order, you get what you get.

Here's my question, though: Why can't those of us who feel weird (at best) about our moms just roll our eyes and move on? Why does watching *Mamma Mia!* make us sob uncontrollably (and not in a fun way)? Why do we still take their calls when chatting with them always makes us feel bad? In other words, why are our moms such a big fucking deal?

Well, scientifically speaking, the game is rigged. We're wired from the start to be such die-hard fans of our caregivers. This default setting is hard to switch off, and it's likely part of the reason you're here, trying to understand your mom and the ways they messed you up.

That's why, in this chapter, we'll get into all the science-backed reasons your mom has such a hold on you. (Not to spoil it, but most of these factors are related to a baby's survival instincts. When you're just trying to make it to your next meal, parents become vital.)

But it's not only biology working against us. We'll also examine the ways society enables moms to move into our brains and stay there for the foreseeable future.

Because mainstream American culture often works to maintain the sanctity of motherhood, the pressure on children to preserve that relationship as adults, no matter how painful, is constant. The culture tells us that you only have one mom, and they love you more than anything. "Life is short," it says, "so make Mother happy while they're here." If you can't, or choose not to, something must be wrong with *you*. You're entitled, you're selfish, or you're ungrateful. (I'm happy to report that's likely not true.)

For better or worse, our moms will never *not* matter to us. And that's a big thing to carry.

WHY YOUR MOM IS SUCH A BIG DEAL

A mom's impact on their children is vast and deep, and can have lasting repercussions. Here's why that is, according to psychologists' research findings.

Moms are often our first line of defense.

You don't get to pick who takes care of you, but as options go, the person who can feed you on demand (historically speaking) is a pretty good one.

"We literally cannot survive without an adult who cares for us. And it's almost always, for a variety of reasons, our biological mother," says psychologist Kathryn Humphreys, PhD, EdM, an associate professor of psychology and human development at Vanderbilt University and director of the Vanderbilt Stress and Early Adversity Laboratory.

That's partly because, for the vast majority of human history, breast milk has been our main food source in the first several months of life, explains Dr. Humphreys. Since most of what babies do is eat, we're bound to spend lots of quality time with the folks who can dispense food from the jump.

Technically speaking, though, there's no concrete reason why moms would be superior caregivers, says Dr. Humphreys. We likely consider moms the default for the reason I just mentioned (boobs), but societal expectations also influence who becomes our primary caregiver, whether you were breastfed or not.

Before you're even born, policies put in place by lawmakers and employers (in the US at least) made it more likely that your mom would be the one caring for you in infancy. Without a nationwide parental leave policy, both parents cannot be fully present with you during those first few weeks or months.

Your brain picks up lots of intel in those early days.

As an infant, you're extra sensitive to information. You take in tons of observations or experiences and turn them into lessons that shape your brain. This is something scientists call developmental plasticity.

In that first month, when you're at your neediest, your brain is about as plastic as it will ever be outside the womb, says Dr. Humphreys. This means the person you hang out with most during that period, often your mom, becomes the most influential. "The relationships we have during those times have an outsized importance relative to the experiences we have later," she adds.

In other words, your mom may have the biggest impact on your life before you even know who they are or how you wound up with them.

Moms and babies may be instinctively obsessed with each other.

A baby's dependency on grownups to stay safe and fed also makes holding mom's attention extra crucial for survival. So, as infants, we do all kinds of adorable and annoying things to get it. Making gurgle-y noises, being very cute, and screaming our faces off are all useful tactics when your life skillset is lacking. This means that, as kids, we intuitively work to get moms to meet our basic needs, if not love us.

Though there are exceptions, caregivers tend to innately find us important too. "Babies are a ton of work—so much work—and it's kind of amazing how many stay alive today," explains Dr. Humphreys. A lot of that can be attributed to medicine, formula, and electricity, but there's also the theory that humans evolved to keep babies alive, she explains.

Take crying, for example. There may be an evolutionary reason why we find it extremely irritating when babies lose their shit. To get some relief, moms (historically speaking) have to solve the thing causing this annoying sound, explains Claudia Brumbaugh, PhD, a social-personality psychologist, researcher studying adult attachment, and professor at Queens College and the Graduate Center of the City University of New York. If true, that theory could explain why caregivers are extremely motivated to feed, change, and snuggle displeased infants.

Babies are sort of like smoke detectors that blare every time they're the least bit uncomfortable. If those cries didn't always feel like an emergency, caregivers might not be as likely to respond.

Our moms can influence our attachment style.

You've probably heard of attachment styles, but just to level-set and deprogram whatever dating or TikTok taught you, allow Dr. Brumbaugh, who also heads up the Attachment, Emotions, and Relationships Lab at the CUNY Graduate Center, to explain: Assuming that your mom was your primary caretaker, your bond with them was your introduction to human relationships. If that's the case, they become your first attachment relationship.

To form an attachment relationship, all you really need is time together, adds Dr. Humphreys. Proximity is what promotes whether or not there is an attachment, not the level of care or how kind someone is.

These attachment relationships begin to form super early in life with what's sometimes called the "initial preattachment" stage, write Omri Gillath, PhD, Gery C. Karantzas, PhD, and R. Chris Fraley, PhD, the authors of *Adult Attachment: A Concise Introduction to Theory and Research.* Within those first couple of months, babies aren't too picky about who's taking care of them. As long as they're being fed, changed, and cuddled, they're mostly good to go.

Then, between two and six months, infants enter the "attachment-in-the-making" stage. This is when babies start getting particular about who's swooping in to meet their needs. For example, the authors write, they might cry until a specific person appears to soothe them. Between months seven and twelve, the "full-blown" or "clear-cut" attachment phase commences, and specific behaviors that define an attachment relationship start to show up. These include seeking out your attachment figure (likely your primary caregiver) and staying near them, avoiding separation from them, reaching out to that person when you're scared or sick, and using them as a "secure base" to return to while exploring your environment, the authors write.

How our primary caregiver treats us during that first year gives us a sense of what we can expect to encounter in other relationships down the road. This idea is based on the theory of internal working models, a thing we'll talk about more in chapter three. What you need to know right now is that your first attachment relationship can become an internal template that you copy and paste onto other relationships, especially in the early days. It can also influence our future expectations of our friends, family, and romantic interests, as well as our beliefs about ourselves.

Let's take a beat to acknowledge how much pressure that puts on moms . . . yikes.

If your mom comes through on most of your baby desires and needs, you're more likely to develop a secure attachment style—the best kind of attachment style, says Dr. Brumbaugh. (Again, more on attachment styles and how your mom influences them in chapter three.) If they don't, well, we'll get into that in chapter four.

Moms help regulate our emotions.

Since we're all born underprepared to face the world or our own feelings, we rely on our caregivers to make us feel better when we're scared, hungry, or just bored. In those early months, they can swoop in to save the day, making us feel more in control.

This trick is called coregulation: a process that allows two people in a relationship, in this case a mom and their baby, to reach an "optimal emotional state," according to a research article published in the journal *Emotion Review*. If you've ever had a bad day, and then called your best friend and felt better afterward, that's coregulation. Same goes if you're extremely sad and your partner gives you a deliciously long hug. You were really upset, and now you feel OK.

In the context of infanthood, caregivers are crucial for helping babies find emotional stability through coregulation. "The belief amongst most people who study early caregiving emotion regulation is that kids don't have the capacity to regulate their emotions on their own for some time," says Dr. Humphreys. Having someone around to borrow chill from is extra important when you're still figuring out what you are and what you're doing here. Eventually, you'll catch on to Emotion Management 101 and need less external support from mom to take the edge off.

That said, it's not like the ability to get it together on your own makes coregulation useless. That's why the best-friend phone call and the hug from your partner still hit the spot. While you'll eventually learn to soothe yourself or find others who can step in when you're feeling out of control, no "I'm good" switch flips on at a certain age.

In fact, Dr. Humphreys says that some research shows that parents can still coregulate with their kids over the phone as they get older—meaning, this aspect of your relationship can be useful for, basically, ever.

Moms show us that we're a big deal.

There might not be anything more powerful for our self-esteem than people doing what we say. When those things happen consistently, we're bound to get the idea that we're very important.

Feed me! Entertain me with your face! Walk me around the room so I may observe my surroundings! You get the idea.

When moms, or any primary caregiver, acts as our humble servant within that first year of life, it supports the belief that our thoughts, feelings, and opinions are worthy of others' attention and action.

That's a perk of the internal working model we talked about earlier. Over time, based on many interactions with our caregivers, we learn that people want to take care of us in a relationship, explains Dr. Brumbaugh. With a foundation of self-worth and self-esteem, we can face the chaos with the sense that we matter. It's like that "I am worthy" affirmation from our Pinterest board/Tumblr/coffee mug has been programmed into our brain. We don't have to just suck it up, apologize for existing, and pack our needs into a box where they don't bother anyone.

Moms teach us how to trust.

Knowing your wants and needs are valid, as they say, is one thing. Believing people are willing to help you achieve contentment is a whole other deal. That's another benefit of a healthy internal working model of attachment. When a baby is well cared for over that first year of life, they learn to trust, says Dr. Brumbaugh. They develop this expectation that *I have needs that deserve to be met, and those needs are met by my people who always come through for me.* It's a lovely perspective on life, and it helps us assume the best in people—within reason.

When you've got this innocent-until-proven-guilty mindset, it's easier to make new connections, trust the barista to get your coffee order right, and avoid a hypervigilant lifestyle.

That trusting nature can also help in romantic relationships. When you believe that people generally want to make you happy, you may feel less skeptical of whoever you're into. You'll trust that they'll do what they say and say what they'll do.

Moms make us feel fail proof.

Trusting those in your immediate circle makes your day-to-day easier, it's true. But a secure working model of attachment also comes complete with the belief that you can survive hard things, says Dr. Brumbaugh.

When your caregiver's response to you as a wee babe is consistent and leaves you feeling content, you start to believe that, even when bad things happen, life usually turns out well (or at least fine). You begin to believe that your social safety net will support you in hard times. You can bank on your brother if you're suddenly homeless after a breakup. You can call your work friends for comfort if you get laid off unexpectedly. The world is way less intimidating when you innately believe that social support is out there for you if and when you need an assist. When your mom straps the golden parachute of secure attachment to your back, jumping into the unknown feels less intimidating.

Moms help us make friends more easily.

There's a concept in social-cognitive psychology called transference—a process in which we project our feelings about past significant others onto a new acquaintance who demonstrates similar traits or qualities, write Dr. Gillath and colleagues in *Adult Attachment.* Those significant others could be an ex (former significant others count), your best friend, and—of course—your mom.

When you're interacting with new people, their personality, the way they look, or their habits can activate our "mental representations" of folks we already have strong connections with, write Dr. Gillath and colleagues.

This means that if you and your mom are securely attached, and you meet someone who reminds you of them, you're more likely to feel safe with that new person. You might even give them the benefit of the doubt.

That's cute! And even better, it can translate to letting your guard down with people you don't know much about—in a good way! "We build relationships by sharing little bits of information about ourselves," explains Dr. Brumbaugh, who's researched transference and interpersonal relationships. "That can seem trivial at first, but it builds to more emotional disclosure and intimate disclosure over time."

So, in theory, your mom (or, again, any primary caretaker) can set you up to be really good at connecting with others. Using that ability can expand your social network and sense of security within those friendships. What power!

Moms make us feel seen.

You know when you're with a close friend and you quote a movie in response to something they say? Then they quote another part of the same movie back to you—and your whole conversation becomes a series of memes from 2014? That process of being seen and responded to accordingly is attunement.

Attunement is the ability to recognize and validate someone's emotional state—someone like a baby. If the baby is excited, an attuned parent responds in an upbeat way. If the baby is scared or sad, the caregiver provides comfort and support. Attunement doesn't mean matching the baby's exact emotion (you wouldn't respond to a sad baby by crying too . . . though you may want to), but the caregiver's reaction should meet the baby where they're at, says Dr. Humphreys. "I think about attunement as feeling understood. That somebody notices me, cares about me, gets my feelings, gets who I am, and values me," she adds.

Thankfully for everyone, your mom doesn't have to be 100 percent attuned to you 100 percent of the time. That would be impossible, honestly. But if you grew up with a mom who was mostly attuned to your feelings, you learn that people notice you, says Dr. Humphreys. They see when you're upset or extremely psyched, and they match your energy in a way that makes you feel understood and cared for. Over time, those experiences become lodged in your brain as a reminder that your people should get you and make you feel important. "I think feeling like you have people in your life who understand you and care about you and validate your feelings is a really fundamental piece of growing up and being emotionally healthy," says Dr. Humphreys.

Moms help us become resilient.

Moms aren't perfectly attuned to their babies all the time; that's impossible. The important part is that they keep trying. In fact, while your mom's attunement to you and your needs is great, miscommunication serves a purpose, too, write Jennifer A. DiCorcia, PhD, and Ed Tronick, PhD, the authors of an article published in the journal *Neuroscience & Biobehavioral Reviews.*

The researchers' theory suggests that when moms misread a baby's cues, like offering a toy instead of a bottle, it makes a stressful situation more intense. But when mom then figures out what their little guy needs and delivers on that, the baby can relax and feel reassured that everything is fine now. That kind of micro-stress tolerance may help babies develop a greater resilience to tough situations in the future, the authors conclude.

Moms are marketed to us.

Aside from the developmental perks, the societal narrative that Moms Are Human Angels Walking Among Us has a major influence too. Mostly perfect mothers are in the cartoons we watched as little kids, the Disney Channel shows we consumed as adolescents, the greeting-card aisle of the drugstore, and the Mother's Day ads from our favorite brunch spot. From the outside, our friends' relationships with their moms might appear as advertised too.

Once you're aware of all that, it's easy to see how the idea of The Mother can become bigger than your experience of having one. Even if our maternal figure leaves us wanting more, the title of "mom" can keep us from seeing this relationship clearly.

Instead of responding to a hurtful relationship in a logical way, we hang on to the dream of what we always wanted our mom to be like. We hold out hope for who they could become. In the meantime, we can just deal, right?

In the end, it might not matter if our mom delivered on all those benefits I just listed or not. Since our culture brands motherhood as an assignment in selfless love and endless unconditional care, of course we want in on that promise! Who wouldn't?

For many of us, this is the biggest reason why our moms matter so much.

We never stop needing our moms.

Parents don't become less important as we get older. We learn to wipe our butts, grab a snack, and dress ourselves, but those skills alone aren't enough to create emotionally mature, confident, trusting grownups.

We still need our primary caregivers to help us feel safe. We need them to establish our sense of belonging. We need their help as we learn to trust. We need them to make us feel important and seen, explains therapist Vienna Pharaon, LMFT, author of *The Origins of You: How Breaking Family Patterns Can Liberate the Way We Live and Love.* "Those things are going to be forever established through the micro and macro moments exchanged between child and parent," she adds. Yep, forever.

As we grow up, we want more time with friends and start telling them our secrets instead of our moms. We might even consider our friends a safe space to vent about mom. Still, attachment theory researchers have found that a majority of the adolescents and teenagers studied are likely to consider their parent—usually their mom—the number one person they count on and the one they want to be with when they're upset.

But wait, there's more. Some attachment research also finds that the importance of our moms continues into adulthood. A few studies (two surveying college kids and one surveying people ages sixteen to ninety) found that—even as people got older, partnered up, or developed super-close friendships—most ranked their mom as their second closest attachment figure. One of those studies found that single people often ranked their moms as number one.

Pharaon says we need our parents to help us navigate the world and our emotions for a really long time. But even after we've reached the point where we *need* our mom, receiving comfort, warmth, and validation from the person who's supposed to understand us more than anyone else in the world still feels good.

WHAT MAKES A "GOOD" MOM?

Not every caregiver is instinctively attuned and sensitive to their children's needs. You're reading a book called *Motherf*cked*, so you've probably got plenty of anecdotal evidence. But it's not just you. Science has the receipts. Dr. Humphreys and her colleague investigated how our current expectations of caregivers (see: mothers) align with expectations of the past. That investigation suggested that, in the scheme of human history, being sensitive to a kid's needs isn't a natural tendency for all moms.

If we zoom way out to see the whole of human existence, it wasn't long ago that roughly half of all kids died before adulthood. So, in theory, keeping an emotional distance from their children could have evolutionary benefits for moms. "If you are a mother of multiple children and half of them are dying, then you might think a little bit differently about the task of raising a child," Dr. Humphreys explains.

She and her colleague write, "Given closer consideration of our evolutionary timescale, in which loss and the experience of adversity were more prevalent than today, it may be that highly sensitive and responsive parenting is not the standard for our species."

That tracks with what Dr. Humphreys sees in her clinical experience today. Some moms do have a natural tendency to be sensitive and in tune with kids, and some don't. The qualities of a good mother aren't necessarily baked into mom DNA. Even if someone isn't inherently excellent at decoding their baby's cries or untangling their middle schooler's drama, what truly counts, notes Dr. Humphreys, is trying to get better at it.

What does "getting better" mean? Studies show that children thrive when their primary caregiver embodies certain qualities. Here are some of the biggies.

Sensitivity

This word encompasses many helpful things parents can do for their kids. Technically speaking, though, maternal sensitivity is a mom's ability to understand and interpret a child's needs and manage them relatively quickly and helpfully, per the *Encyclopedia of Evolutionary Psychological Science.*

Studies suggest that when your mom prioritizes your needs in infancy, you're more likely to get in on all those benefits we just talked about, like trust, self-esteem, and more.

Acceptance

Acceptance means recognizing who someone is and adjusting your expectations for them based on that. When your caregiver accepts you as you are—not who they wish you were—it helps you see that you're valuable and important. Your mom's acceptance proves you're good enough as is.

Stimulation

We haven't talked about this much, but parents impact how we think, learn, and understand the world, not just how we feel. If moms create stimulating environments for their babies—where they can see new things, hear new words, and flex their brain by using other senses like touch and smell—they set kids up to develop better problem-solving and decision-making skills in the future, says Dr. Humphreys.

THE LEGACY OF THE MOTHER

The ways our moms can set us up for success are almost endless. How they treat us as kids can get embedded into the way we see the world, relationships, and ourselves, and this perspective has a lasting impact on us as we grow up (more on that in chapter three).

In short, moms' time, attention, and consistent care can help us develop into emotionally mature, resilient, confident, trusting, and friendly people. It may also reduce our risk of developing various mental health conditions, as several studies suggest.

The way moms are sold to us as kids and beyond influences us too. When you assume your mom loves you more than anything, it's easy to give them the benefit of the doubt, even when they don't come through. The idea that moms are important makes them important.

Now that we know a little more about why moms matter and what ideal mom behavior looks like, let's discuss what gets in the way of that.

CHAPTER 2

Why Some Moms Struggle to Mom

In a perfect world, your mom's consistent, warm, attuned care will help transform you from a worm into a securely attached, trusting, happy, emotionally regulated person who feels loved and important.

But we don't live in a perfect world, and for those of us who don't have a healthy relationship with our moms, the promises of the close maternal relationship outlined in chapter one can feel unfamiliar. We're not running around feeling indestructible and reassured that things will probably work out. We're still second-guessing whether people like us and if we're worthy of our goals. We're unconvinced that our people will have our backs. We might not even be sure that we matter.

That's because, unfortunately, receiving quality care and attention from your mom requires that they have the physical, emotional, and mental capabilities to offer them. Sometimes they don't have these—or, if they do, they may lack the desire to offer them.

Most mothers want to do what's best for their kids. They want to help us become good people who do good things and feel generally good about ourselves. However, when your mom's attention is focused on something more pressing (which could be *a lot* of things), there's less of a spotlight to shine on your needs.

Many factors can make healthy mom-ing a challenging task. Without money, time, supportive friends or family, information, and coping skills, parenting can get real dysfunctional, real fast. Add in things like trauma, cultural expectations, or mental health conditions, and you've got a child-rearing situation that kind of sucks for everyone involved. Good intentions and high hopes are not always enough to overcome the challenges moms face. And unfortunately, the consequences of your mom's shortcomings can harm you and your relationship with them for the foreseeable future.

If all this makes you feel a little hopeless or like your relationship with your mom was cursed from the start, I get it. Still, identifying the possible sources of your mom's dysfunction may ease the discomfort. By understanding the factors that influence her special brand of parenting, you can find empathy for her, reframe tough memories, and reassess your narrative. You might also feel less reactive to her chronically unhinged behavior. She's messy, but there's probably a reason why, and understanding that something completely unrelated to you is likely behind her behavior can make you feel a smidge better.

NINE CLASSIC MOM BLOCKERS

There are roughly one kajillion things that make it harder for moms to show up in a healthy way. Some of those are within their control, some are not. Here are a few of the most common reasons why moms don't end up doing their best.

1. They didn't want or weren't ready to have a baby.

Not all people who get pregnant want to be pregnant. This is not breaking news. And because getting pregnant doesn't necessarily reprogram a person's brain to make them a loving, involved parent, sometimes unwanted pregnancies can turn into unwanted children. When that happens, the relationship between those moms and their kids can suffer.

In one study, researchers surveyed nearly five thousand couples with newborns. They also followed up with the parents at various points in their kids' childhoods to check in on the family dynamics and the child's development. An analysis of that data found that when a mom reported her pregnancy was unintended, there was a higher risk of her being "psychologically aggressive"—that is, shouting and swearing at her child—during the three-year check in. There was also a higher risk of her neglecting her child.

While that survey focused more on low-income parents and isn't nationally representative, other studies suggest that when parents plan to have a child, they provide that child with better care.

2. Their reasons for having a baby weren't great.

Even when a mom plans to have a baby, sometimes her goals in having one is unrealistic, which can leave her disappointed once the baby arrives.

As part of their research at the Vanderbilt Stress and Early Adversity Laboratory, Kathryn Humphreys and her team often ask expectant mothers why they wanted to have a baby. Not everyone can pinpoint the exact reason, but a few themes tend to come up. For some, babies are an important aspect of their religion. Having kids may also be an expectation of their community or family. In my experience as a mental health editor and reporter, any mental health pro will tell you that making a personal choice based on others' preferences doesn't usually turn out well. And when that decision is whether to have a baby or not, the stakes are pretty high.

Similarly, Dr. Humphreys says moms-to-be sometimes have ideas of what this baby will do for them. They want to have a kid so there will be someone to take care of them when they're older. Or they think a child will fill an emotional need, like providing unconditional love and support. Yeah, their kid might go on to do both of those things, but expectations like that put way too much pressure on the baby, who didn't apply for those jobs. If the kiddo doesn't deliver, mom can be disappointed. It's hard to say exactly how that could impact the way she shows up as a parent, but it doesn't seem ideal.

3. Their energy is spent.

Like all people, moms only have so much physical, mental, and emotional energy to give. Plot that energy as a pie chart; with each stressor, another slice gets claimed. Clinical psychologist Jenny Tzu-Mei Wang, PhD, author of *Permission to Come Home: Reclaiming Mental Health as Asian Americans*, describes this as a fracturing of energy (which sounds way cooler than my pie chart), but the idea is the same: More life demands leave moms less energy to spare.

That's true for physical stressors too. Anyone who's experienced a hangover after the age of twenty-two knows how difficult it is to be your best self when you're exhausted. Whatever the source of physical depletion, it forces you to devote most of your energy to staying upright, awake, and accomplishing the bare minimum. There's nothing left for tasks like filtering thoughts before they become words. Responding thoughtfully or maturely to someone's attitude is also a nonstarter. Any minor inconvenience could cause a meltdown. That experience holds true for moms too. Having a kid doesn't make being a person in a body any easier.

Whether you know this firsthand as a parent or not, your physical and mental capacities are intertwined. When just getting through the day in one piece sucks up your bandwidth, your emotional abilities take a hit.

Things like chronic illness, physical limitations, and substance use can certainly hamper how moms show up for their kids. But those aren't the only stressors that make healthy parenting a challenge. A bank account in despair could mean working more hours, taking on multiple jobs, or disappearing into the job search process. Any of these could keep moms from being mentally present for Pikachu impressions or physically present for middle-school graduations.

Of course, making money isn't the only type of time suck for moms. A tale as old as time: Moms take on the majority of life chores and child-rearing, even if they have day jobs. When so many big-deal responsibilities fall on one person, important stuff is bound to get neglected. While said stuff could be a sink full of dishes, it could also be parent-teacher conferences or deep conversations about feelings.

Like money and time, community is another scarce resource that supports healthy parenting, says Minaa B., LMSW, author of *Owning Our Struggles: A Path to Healing and Finding Community in a Broken World.*

Friends, family, and other members of the community enable moms to take a breather, vent, and feel less alone. Like anyone, moms need a damn break—even if that means complaining on the phone with the bathroom door locked during nap time. "Community care is childcare," says Minaa B. "If it's literally just a caregiver or even a caregiver and their partner doing the mental, emotional, and physical work of taking care of that child, the lack of communal support can wear the body down," she explains.

That can cause mental health challenges like stress and anxiety, which impact a mom's ability to parent effectively, Minaa B. notes. Amid unrelenting stress, it's tough to keep calm enough to carry on with kids.

Being present and sensitive, and reciprocating childhood enthusiasm, can easily fall through the cracks when moms are physically drained. From what I can tell, it doesn't make being a parent to adult kids any easier either.

4. They're emotionally unequipped.

This feels like a good time to get into emotional maturity. Chances are you've heard of her (or her nemesis, emotional *immaturity*).

The American Psychological Association (APA) describes emotional maturity as "a high and appropriate level of emotional control and expression," in contrast to emotional immaturity, which the APA calls "a tendency to express emotions without restraint or disproportionately to the situation."

So, people who are more emotionally developed are aware of their feelings and able to express them appropriately, depending on who they're with and what's happening around them.

To be clear, being emotionally mature doesn't mean packing up your feelings and tossing them into *Aladdin*'s cave of wonders. Instead, it requires using empathy and context clues to determine how you show up in the moment. Emotionally mature people crash out too; they just do it in a time and place that's safe for them and everyone else involved. Also, emotional maturity exists on a spectrum ranging from extremely immature to extremely mature, as measured by the Emotional Maturity Scale (EMS).

The EMS has been used to measure emotional maturity in several scientific studies investigating things like the emotional maturity of young adults online, adolescents, and lonely college students. Traits on the immature end of the EMS include reactivity, feelings of inferiority, lying, and pessimism. On the mature side of the spectrum, you'll find emotional stability, social adaptability, contentment, and independence.

Everyone's baseline of emotional maturity falls somewhere between those two points, but we can backslide depending on the day. When we're stressed, scared, tired, overwhelmed, or triggered, it's easy to slip into emotionally immature behaviors, writes Whitney Goodman, LMFT, creator of Calling Home, a community (and podcast) for adults who want to improve their family relationships and end generational patterns of dysfunction. That said, even when everything is going well, some people are more emotionally equipped to take life on than others.

Moms also fall somewhere on that spectrum (perhaps you're too aware of this). While your mom's baseline can be influenced by her nature and how she was raised, so can experiences like trauma, abuse, and neglect—especially if she never sought resources to work through the emotional repercussions.

Your mom's emotional maturity level might be super apparent when they're going through a rough patch or having a bad day, but it can also reveal itself in everyday interactions.

Here's a scenario for you: Say your mom is coming to visit you for a fun little vacay. She arrives, you play tourists for the weekend, and she's off. Then, a week or so later, during the workday, she sends you a text. Your childhood cat has died. More specifically, after a long illness, your mom has made the difficult decision to put kitty to rest. You're obviously devastated. RIP, buddy. Thank you for the memories.

A minute later, your mom texts again. This time, she sends a photo of herself with a kitten. She adopted a new one, seemingly seconds after its predecessor's demise. "Wait, what?" you ask. The rebound from last rites to "New cat; who's this?" seems to have been a matter of minutes.

Your mom admits that, not long before her frolic in your city, she put your OG cat down. But you guys had plans, and she didn't want to kill the vibe of her trip with sad news. Instead, she planned to tell you later, at a more opportune time. You know, like a Tuesday afternoon while you're in the office, the most convenient place to get very sad, unexpected news, obviously.

Shall we count the emotional immaturity touchpoints?

1. Prioritizing her own footloose and fancy-free weekend ahead of being a source of emotional support
2. Choosing to tell you bad news at a time that's best for her (a.k.a. after trading in the old model for a new one and wanting to tell someone)
3. Not giving you any time to process that sad moment before completely moving on

An emotionally mature mom, on the other hand, might have decided to tell you in person when she arrived and made herself available to help you through the loss, even if it overlapped with her PTO. She may have taken you out for ice cream to help you feel better (aw!).

Or, even if she waited until she returned home to share the news, she could have called you at a time she knew you'd be someplace comfortable and private and offered emotional support over the phone. Or! She could have texted you saying, "Are you somewhere you can talk?" and then waited for you to get there and call her back. So many options!

Whatever form it takes, the emotionally mature mom's approach comes from a place of thoughtfulness and consideration. She considers your feelings and needs alongside her own. The emotionally immature mom . . . does not.

5. They don't know how to cope.

A coping mechanism is a conscious or unconscious adjustment to alleviate tension or anxiety in a stressful situation, according to the APA.

Coping mechanisms help people navigate triggers or get through tough moments in a healthy way. Individuals might seek support from community, a trusted friend, or a therapist. They might engage in grounding techniques that help them get centered. They might start doing yoga or reading self-help books. They might get really into astrology or breathwork. So cute! So healthy!

However, when the way someone deals with tension becomes more harmful than helpful, those coping mechanisms become maladaptive.

Maladaptive coping mechanisms include drinking, drugs, yelling, toxic positivity (maintaining that things are fine when they're clearly not), overspending, compulsive lying, isolating yourself, hoarding, and physical violence. And there are many, many more where those came from.

Whitney Goodman explains that when people don't have the resources—like money, time, or emotional bandwidth—to find healthy ways to feel safe in tumultuous situations, they're more likely to reach for maladaptive coping mechanisms. And you know what eats up money, time, and emotional bandwidth? Children!

On top of that, raising kiddos can make parents think about their own childhoods. Parenting can become a challenging minefield of triggers to navigate, and so moms may find themselves in a maladaptive coping spiral out of self-preservation, says Goodman.

Sometimes that means attempting to use maladaptive tools for good. For example, a mom might use maladaptive coping mechanisms to feel closer or bond with their kids. They might drink (see: wine moms) to make time together feel more fun. You know, they're "not a regular mom" and all that.

Other times, maladaptive coping mechanisms enable moms to get some distance from their kids, says Goodman. That could look like scrolling to escape uncomfortable quality time or putting up a wall because mom thinks their kids are better off without them.

6. They're dealing with trauma.

Trauma can get in the way of moms showing up as their best parental selves more generally too.

When people experience events they can't cope with (see: trauma), it can shape how they express emotions and change how they connect with people. That's even more likely if they never sought out treatment or support to process what happened and grow from it, says Dr. Wang. A breakup, job loss, illness, or other major setback can make managing whatever comes next harder. That's true for everyone, including moms.

A study by Dr. Humphreys and her colleagues showed that pregnant women who experienced life-altering events during their pregnancy, like the sudden death of a loved one, a car accident, jail time, assault, or divorce, were more likely to have "distorted representations" of their future baby. These distorted representations could show up as internal inconsistencies in how the mom thinks about their future child ("I know babies cry, but I expect mine will be different"), unrealistic expectations for their baby ("My child will never have tantrums if I just love them enough"), or a preoccupation with their own anxieties or stressors ("This baby will finally give my life meaning"). They found the same was true for pregnant women who experienced stressful situations during their childhood.

In theory, these kinds of mindsets could negatively impact how those moms go on to care for their kids (or don't) once they're born. Previous research suggests that distorted representations are associated with less sensitive parenting and insecure attachment in infants. Still, it's not like these moms are going out of their way to be jerks. They're victims of their circumstances too.

The same idea could apply to moms dealing with domestic violence. People in abusive relationships dedicate so much mental and emotional energy to safely navigating that dynamic. It takes a lot of conscious and unconscious decision making and threat assessment to keep everyone safe. That can make calmly responding to kids' day-to-day needs more challenging, says Dr. Wang.

Intergenerational trauma can also show up in how your mom moms. This kind of trauma happens when family members experience an event (like a natural disaster) or an ongoing situation (like slavery or forced migration) and aren't able to process what happened and/or heal from it, Dr. Wang explains. Such trauma can affect the way they show up as caregivers, creating unhelpful patterns that are perpetuated through generations.

Intergenerational or not, trauma that's left unhealed can cause people to go through life on high alert. At any moment, their fight-or-flight response could be triggered and send them spiraling. Obviously, that's not a great foundation for raising kids, which is triggering in itself, says Dr. Wang. The combo of unresolved trauma and nonstop triggers can weaken emotional regulation and communication skills, key components of emotional maturity.

Since people respond to adversity in different ways, experiencing trauma doesn't always result in failing as a parent. For example, some caregivers realize that it wasn't fun to be ignored by their parents. Then, when they have kids, they make a particular effort to be supportive and emotionally available. Dr. Wang says that's a thing. It just doesn't always work out that way.

7. They have an insecure attachment style.

Growing up without healthy examples of what it means to be a parent can make becoming one more challenging, says Minaa B. In her experience, moms who established a secure attachment with their caregiver as a child are more likely to do the same for their kids.

That could be because they know the importance of sensitive, attuned, and consistent care. "I do believe that when parents come from a secure attachment base, where they experienced a sense of care, bonding, and emotional and psychological safety, they can be a little more in tune with their emotions," Minaa B. explains. When these securely attached parents give birth, they tend to have a stronger parenting skillset, making it easier for them to develop a secure attachment with their own child.

It's also possible that a mom's secure attachment to their mother equips them with greater resilience when facing the overwhelming task of raising a baby. "Resilience allows moms to approach parenting from a lens of, *This is difficult, but I can find ways to manage it,*" explains Minaa B. Without that mindset, she adds, moms find it harder to develop the tools or coping skills needed to deal with their kids. For some caregivers, a lack of resilience can make the challenges of parenting feel like a personal attack.

While I didn't find any studies suggesting that securely attached moms go on to have securely attached babies (who later have their own securely attached kiddos), the theory makes sense. Plus, there *is* some research correlating a mother's general attachment style to their relationship with their children. For example, one study found that moms who had an avoidant attachment style (a kind of insecure attachment style) didn't feel as close to their preschool-aged kids as securely attached moms did.

8. Their mental health got in the way.

Speaking of emotional challenges, nothing comes for emotional stability like a mental health condition.

Just so we're all on the same page, a mental health condition is a diagnosable disorder listed in the ever-evolving bible of mental health disorders, the revised version of the fifth-edition *Diagnostic and Statistical Manual of Mental Disorders (DSM-5-TR)*. Any mental health condition, whether you have an official diagnosis or not, can make life more taxing. To even receive a diagnosis, many people need to experience symptoms of their condition for months—even years. While treatment can certainly help manage those symptoms and the fallout, the condition is often with you till the end.

I'm laying this out in the hope that we can all agree that mental health disorders are incredibly tough to navigate. They take time and money to treat, and the path to feeling better isn't always linear.

Unfortunately for moms (who are already tasked with the majority of baby handling), mental health challenges can stifle the hell out of good intentions. Depression is a solid example. Depressive disorders come with "sad, empty, or irritable mood, accompanied by related changes that significantly affect the individual's capacity to function," according to the *DSM-5-TR*. Those symptoms, which can last from two weeks to two years at a time, can make even the idea of getting out of bed physically and mentally exhausting.

When you're struggling to take care of yourself, looking out for others can be very difficult, says Dr. Wang. From her clinical experience, untreated depression can get in the way of a parent's ability to read kids' cues (especially babies') and respond in an emotionally regulated way. They might not even be able to show up at all.

Depression may also impact a parent's ability to see the world from their kid's perspective. That skill is called empathy, and one study published by Dr. Humphreys and her colleagues found that parents' depressive symptoms were associated with lower levels of empathy for their toddlers—even lower than their empathy for adult strangers.

Empathizing with a kid is often the first step in helping them through whatever they're dealing with, especially when they're tiny and helpless.

If moms don't get why their kid is crying or don't feel concerned, they could be less likely to do something about it.

Not surprisingly, postpartum depression can also make being a quality mom extra hard. One review of research suggests that moms who showed signs of depression at the time of childbirth displayed less closeness, warmth, and sensitivity with their baby. The same review also reported that moms with depression were less emotionally available for their kiddo during the first year.

Likewise, anxiety disorders can change how people see the world and the way they exist in it. This type of mental health condition, per the *DSM-5-TR*, is one in which a person's excessive fear and anxiety affects how they function.

For example, people with generalized anxiety disorder are overly anxious or worried more days than not for at least six months. Those worries feel out of control and can result in symptoms like sleep struggles, trouble concentrating, fatigue, and restlessness, according to the *DSM-5-TR*.

Whether that anxiety is a legit diagnosis or not, living with anxiety means existing in a state of fear. So moms who are chronically worried may instill certain anxieties in their kids, says Minaa B. When moms feel helpless and scared, she explains, their kid may feel the same.

Also, a caregiver's anxiety can impact the way they raise their child, explains Minaa B. Even if they don't realize they're doing it, moms who go through life feeling consistently scared and unsafe can project their fears onto their kids. Children can pick up on that, adds Minaa B. Sometimes that results in kids taking on the caregiver role, attempting to protect their parent from the stuff they're scared of, she explains.

The one type of mental health issue that kept coming up in my interviews with therapists, psychologists, and researchers was personality disorders. These conditions are the basis of many a Reddit thread, and they're one of the most stigmatized mental health disorders out there. That's likely because they're characterized by deviation from societal norms and symptoms that can get in the way of showing empathy and compassion, being sensitive, and having self-awareness.

Take narcissistic personality disorder (NPD). While the internet loves to label every bad ex, parent, and high school nemesis as just another self-obsessed narcissist, the disorder is more complicated than that.

To be clinically diagnosed with NPD, a person needs to have five of the nine official criteria, which include an exaggerated sense of self-importance, a sense of entitlement, a need for admiration, and a lack of empathy. People with NPD often take advantage of others to benefit themselves. They might also believe that others are envious of them. Whatever the symptoms, they have to be present pretty much constantly, or in what the *DSM-5-TR* calls a pervasive pattern.

Since parenting requires a ton of self-sacrifice, sensitivity, and empathy—the traits people with this condition lack—it can be extremely hard for moms with NPD to be quality caregivers, says Minaa B.

Whether they *want* to be the best parent ever or not, "that grandiose sense of self can create a disconnect," she explains. "They have a hard time being in tune with the emotional needs of their child because they're only concerned about their own."

Yeah, not ideal. Just to clarify, people with NPD, including parents, can still understand what other people are feeling to some degree (that's called cognitive empathy). The problem is that they're unwilling to recognize the feelings or needs of others, per the *DSM-5-TR*.

We should also take a sec to chat about undiagnosable mental health conditions, what some are now calling a high-functioning situation. Though it's not an official term, it means someone is experiencing many of the symptoms of specific disorders like depression, anxiety, or borderline personality disorder, but doesn't meet the criteria for a diagnosis. Minna B. says that any kind of behavior that's rooted in a mental health issue can affect parenting. Your mom doesn't need an official diagnosis for their mental health issues to affect how they treat you.

9. They didn't know better.

This sounds like a poor excuse in a time when the internet exists, but it's a fact: It's hard for parents who don't know better to do better.

Sometimes that ignorance stems from their upbringing. The way our parents were raised can perpetuate harmful coping mechanisms and ideas about what's acceptable and what's not.

A mom who was beaten for misbehaving might assume corporal punishment is a solid teaching tool. Another mom who was shamed for crying or voicing an opinion might do the same to their kid. Likewise, if their parents never held themselves accountable or demonstrated emotional maturity, those are more lessons lost. For example, if your grandparents went off when your mom made a mistake or did something mischievous, your mom also might think screaming is an acceptable response—and that there's no need to apologize for it.

You get the idea. Minaa B. says these issues may all be part of a larger system failure: a lack of psychoeducation. In her experience, this is often the common denominator in dysfunctional families. When parents don't realize how important their role is or what's required to nurture a child, especially in those early years, it's difficult to change course.

When moms have more of that intel, it's easier for them to spot the problems with their own upbringing. They can think critically about how they're parenting now and choose to act differently, Minaa B. explains.

They can take a step back, realize their actions aren't helpful, and try to do better.

WHAT DO I DO WITH ALL THIS?

If this chapter has left you feeling like "Oh my god, this is bleak as fuck," same. And we've barely scratched the surface here.

Your reaction to these origin stories might also include guilt. Once you've acknowledged ye olde *Hurt people hurt people* adage, it's normal to feel bad about feeling bad. This chapter is not a get-out-of-accountability-quick scheme for your mom, though. Not in this house. You don't have to excuse your mom's hurtful behavior—even if it was rooted in an equally messed-up experience. Unfortunately, moms who did not set out to be an asshole can still become one. That's on them.

I'm not saying your mom's painful experiences don't matter. They do. Empathizing with them helps you see your mom as a complex person who's worthy of compassion like anyone else. That perspective is a kindness to them. But putting yourself in your mom's shoes isn't *for* them. It's for you. Thinking about all the scenarios that could have led to their problematic behavior can free you from blame, change your response to their rude behavior, and enable you to set healthy boundaries (wow, we have so much to get to).

As children, who are egocentric by nature, we tend to blame ourselves for how our parents treat us. It's just a side effect of being a kid, says Dr. Wang. We put the onus on ourselves or believe stories we've been told: We were too much to handle, we didn't listen, we were too sensitive, we *wanted* to be a caregiver for our parents or siblings. Whatever the story, we often make the state of this relationship our fault, which weighs on our self-esteem and self-worth, adds Dr. Wang.

By considering what else could get in the way of healthy parent–child relationships, you can see that it probably wasn't about you. Even if you were the perfect kid (not a thing, by the way), your mom wouldn't have been any different.

Empathy can also soften your reactions to your mom when they pull a dick move. Instead of lashing out, you can pause and reflect on where their behavior might be coming from. Even if you're just guessing, you get to decide whether or not you react, says Dr. Wang. If their behavior isn't about you, maybe it has less power over you? It could happen.

When you step back to consider the experiences that made your mom who they are, you can also spot their shortcomings: where they missed opportunities to grow, seek support, or gain self-awareness. If those choices still affect how they act today, you can choose to protect yourself, says Minaa B. "You can have compassion for your mom, knowing what they've dealt with, but also recognize that you deserve empathy too."

You! Deserve! Empathy! Too! Let's all like, follow, and subscribe to that one.

At the risk of sounding all "Pull yourself up by your bootstraps, son!" people do have free will. If anyone wants to be a more sensitive, empathetic, emotionally mature member of society—and/or parent—they can take steps to get there.

So, while it may be harder for some to change—especially those with limited resources and other systematic obstacles—we're not necessarily doomed by our circumstances.

That's an important lesson to take into the next chapter: When you notice a problem, you can do something about it. Since you're here reading this, I'm guessing that you already have.

As kids, we're likely unaware that hardship, society, trauma, and mental health struggles already may have put Mother through some shit—and the repercussions could impact life as we know it. But once we get the sense that something is off, whether it's directly related to our mom or not, a lot of us wind up talking to a therapist. And the stuff that comes up . . . well, it often ties back to our mothers.

CHAPTER 3

Why Moms Always Come Up in Therapy

In chapter one, we learned about all the ways our caregivers can set us up for success. Thanks mostly to attachment theory, our parents have the power to be a major positive influence on how we see ourselves, other people, and our relationships. But we've also seen, per chapter two, how our moms' mental health struggles, trauma, and life in general can keep them from becoming straight-A parents.

Turns out, all the opportunities moms have to set us up for success can also become opportunities for them to let us down. And these letdowns create a rocky foundation for us to build a life on.

The most obvious collateral damage of your mom's parenting mistakes is your relationship with her: how you view each other and interact, the things you don't say to each other, the stuff you fight about. That's not all though. The way she mommed you can also bubble to the surface in the rest of your life.

You're probably familiar with the trope that all our personal failings, challenges, and emotional shortcomings can be traced back to our family of origin. It's an idea closely associated with "whiny" millennials (a group with which I am affiliated) and their mental health.

This stereotype exists for a reason, says therapist Vienna Pharaon. Your mom's history and experiences affect how she shows up as *your* mom, and your history and experiences with her affect how *you* show up as an adult.

Because this track is so played out, singing along can feel cliché. You might even avoid connecting the dots between your current struggles and your mom because it seems dramatic or self-centered.

Still, Pharaon explains, regarding your relationship with your mom, "It already happened. It existed. It's a part of your story. Your job is to name it." Understanding this relationship provides a huge chunk of information that can shed light on the way you see the world, your unhelpful patterns, how you show up in your relationships, and more.

Whether you're feeling some kind of way about this or not, acknowledging your mom's impact isn't the end of the story. It's just the step that comes before acceptance, finding your sense of agency, and making changes that shift life for the better. (Trust, we'll get to that in part two.)

In the meantime, you will not be surprised to hear that I relate to this blame-your-mom narrative and the resistance to it.

For those who skipped the intro to this book, I used to work at *Cosmopolitan*. When I started in 2017 as a senior editor, I was so proud to plant my ass in that seat. As a paid subscriber to the 2010s' girl-boss era, I'd usually show up at 9 AM and leave at 7:30 PM. Every day for the first year, I wore a bracelet that said "hustle" as a reminder to suck it up and work. This was the big leagues. I am a try-hard.

But despite positive feedback from my team, I never felt like I was one of them. Everyone was smart, funny, and, most importantly, cool—especially the people who sat near me. Naturally, I took it as a personal failure every time I didn't know the writer, restaurant, or show they name-dropped.

In my mind, the only reason I wasn't aware of that Bushwick restaurant or the new *New York Times* feature or the latest episode of *Big Mouth* was because I was an ignorant loser. It wasn't that most of my brain cells were dedicated to proving myself. It wasn't that I did not live in Brooklyn or watch animated series. Rather, I should've known all the cool things cool people knew or else I was not cool, and, therefore, trash.

I wanted to make friends at *Cosmo*, but I'd avoid chiming into casual conversations with the team—lest the attention turn toward me and set my face aflame. It was easier to tell myself no one cared what I had to say than drop an "OMG, I know what you mean," turn bright red, stumble over my words, and go back to my desk mentally replaying the last thing I said for hours. A compliment would fuck me up in the same way. Any attention was too much to handle.

Office chats aside, this must-be-perfect kind of anxiety got in the way of doing big parts of my job. As I said, I couldn't get through a pitch meeting without struggling to read or breathe—usually both.

It wasn't my first anxiety era. Years before, the spirals started showing up in my post-college friendships. I'd tell a story at dinner and become highly aware of my face, hands, and words. It was like watching Ring-cam footage of myself while I talked or listened to someone else. *Does my face look like I'm paying attention right now? Did I mispronounce that word? Where did she grow up again? Can she tell I don't remember? Oh my god, I just missed what she said.*

I get that this inner monologue sounds trivial, but my body responded to it like a death threat.

I often doubted that my best friends even liked me that much. I wondered if something was medically wrong with my brain. Though I'd heard of social anxiety (MentalHealthTok was not a thing at that point), I didn't know why I struggled to be comfortable in my skin, but I knew I was the problem.

Annnnnnd that's pretty much everything I told my therapist when I started seeing her. Maybe you recall this story from the intro: A few months into our sessions, she asked why I worried so much about my boss, coworkers, cool strangers, or friends thinking I was weird or awkward. After weeks of repeating things like "No one wants to be the Phoebe Buffay of their friend group!" I heard myself say, "I don't want to be like my mom." And then came the tissues.

My therapist: "Ah, yeah, that seems like something."

Thus, my *Motherf*cked* journey commenced.

SIGNS YOUR MOM'S DRAMA IS AFFECTING YOUR LIFE

I realize my brand of anxiety and negative self-talk might be different from what you're dealing with right now. It might even seem like no big deal in comparison. That said, I bring you my neurosis as an example of how our relationship with our moms seeps into other compartments of our adult lives, taking us down like the *Titanic*.

As adults, it feels like we're mostly in charge of how we live, love, and respond to challenges, but we could be wrong. Decades of psychological research have concluded that relationships with our caregivers—again, often our moms—can affect the way we function as grown people. Yeah, I hate this as much as you do.

A lot of this, as I mentioned, has to do with attachment theory. There's also the fact that, from infancy, we're watching everything our moms say and do—or don't say and don't do. We're taking notes whether we realize it or not. Those observations often turn into unconscious habits, patterns, and coping strategies that, if left unchecked, can fuck us up in the long run.

Whether you've done this type of therapeutic excavation or not, I know I'm not the only one out here feeling like two kids stacked on top of each other in a trench coat. And there's a good chance your mom contributed to at least some of the seemingly unrelated challenges you're facing now.

Your relationships don't feel cozy or comfortable.

Feel like no one gets you, everyone's hanging out without you, and the people you date are always unreliable? One of the biggest reasons so many of our adult relationship struggles can be traced back to our dynamic with our moms is because of the oversized role our moms play in our baby lives.

Our maternal relationship sets the tone for how most of us see other people, relationships, and ourselves in those early years and sometimes in adulthood (more on that in a sec).

But how? As we discussed in chapter one, attachment theory makes parents a really big deal from the start. And because mothers are a primary source of food and comfort for many babies, most develop an attachment relationship with their moms.

Attachment relationships are those in which you prefer to stay physically close to someone, rely on them as a source of safety, and use them as a "secure base" from which to return to as you explore the world, write Dr. Gillath and her co-authors in *Adult Attachment: A Concise Introduction to Theory and Research.*

When they're our first example of human connection, moms can inadvertently teach us what we should expect from other people and relationships, and what others expect of us. They also teach us about our worth. All of those lessons are learned via the way we're treated—in other words, our early attachment experiences.

As we covered a couple of chapters ago, babies are constantly taking in how caregivers respond to their cries, nonsense sounds, and facial expressions. In other words, they're picking up on how their handlers handle them.

Per attachment theory, babies compile this valuable data to develop ideas, thoughts, attitudes, expectations, and beliefs about themselves and everyone else, to form what psychologists call "internal working models." Think of these as a pair of goggles strapped to your little face, altering how you see the world.

If your mom was consistent, warm, empathetic, and attuned to you as a baby, the world and the people in it are more likely to appear nice and rosy in those early years. As a result, you're also more likely to feel confident—ready to crush childhood—and believe that you matter. In addition, you may expect people to be relatively trustworthy and willing to help when you need it. These are all classic side effects of a secure internal working model of attachment (also known as a secure attachment style). It's the best working model of attachment money cannot buy.

Of course, not everyone gets that first-class, King Baby experience. When a primary caregiver, such as your mom, doesn't respond quickly, appropriately, or in a way that makes you feel seen—and does so over and over again—you can develop an insecure working model of attachment or an insecure attachment style.

When that happens, your ideas, thoughts, attitudes, expectations, and beliefs about yourself and everyone else are less warm and fuzzy. Your internal working model may lead you to believe you're unworthy of love and attention. You might assume that people are untrustworthy and you're on your own.

As you get older, those early attachment experiences can influence how you show up in your childhood friendships. Though the research is mixed, there's evidence that children who are securely attached to their caregivers have stronger interpersonal skills, like empathy and emotional understanding, which helps them make and keep friends. Those friendships can help set the groundwork for healthy adult attachment relationships too.

But let's clear something up really quick. Yes, moms set the vibe for how we see ourselves and other people as littles. However, despite what you've heard on TikTok, that early attachment style isn't necessarily locked in.

Several decades of research say that, even if our moms treated us like trash, future experiences with teachers, friends, mentors, and partners can undo the damage. This helps us become more secure, sure of ourselves, and trusting of other people over time. Yay for that!

However, the reason I'm still out here talking about early attachment is because there's a nugget of association between your childhood relationship with your mom and the way you function in relationships as an adult. It's small, but it isn't zero.

For example, in one study that followed participants for more than twenty-five years, researchers found that individuals who had a closer emotional bond with their moms as children and adolescents were more social, caring, and affectionate adults. They were also less likely to avoid emotional closeness in their relationships (see: avoidant attachment, a type of insecure attachment).

To be fair, that correlation was strongest in people who carried certain genes. However, another study following kids and their families for eighteen years had similar results: Children whose moms were sensitive to their needs were less likely to have an avoidant attachment style at the age of eighteen. The same study also found that when moms were less responsive and available to their kids as they got older, those kids were more likely to become avoidantly attached eighteen-year-olds.

So, if your mom sort of "let go and let God" after your infancy, it can make a dent in your psyche. When that dent comes in the form of avoidant attachment, you might feel uncomfortable relying on others or opening up to people. You might not love it when others get vulnerable with you. That's why an avoidant attachment style can make emotional intimacy with close friends or partners a real challenge.

The results of that eighteen-year study also suggest that adults whose moms experienced more depressive symptoms over time were more likely to have an *anxious* attachment style, which like avoidant attachment can also mess with your relationships in adulthood. Anxious attachment often shows up as a fear that others won't be there when you need them or that you're not worthy of love. It can also impact your self-esteem, says Dr. Brumbaugh.

The study authors found that when moms reported experiencing symptoms of depression when their kids were little, those kids were more likely to be anxiously attached by the time they were of legal age to vote. Same goes if the moms' symptoms worsened over time.

If we lose our mom's attention, presence, compassion, gentleness, or warmth, we notice. So, part of the reason those childhood experiences with our mom infiltrate our adult relationships and how we see ourselves could be that we make their behavior about us.

As kids, if we see that our moms are sad all the time, don't have time for us, don't pay attention to us, or otherwise distance themselves from us, we can easily internalize it, says Pharaon. We tell ourselves, consciously or not, *If my mom doesn't love me or choose me, who will?*

When that idea sticks with you through childhood, you may start to look for evidence that you're not worthy of other people's time and attention. If you find it, you risk confirmation bias–ing your way to an insecure attachment style as an adult.

While insecure attachment doesn't damn you to an eternity of hissing at people from a dark alley, it could make life harder. You might be less likely to give people the benefit of the doubt, feel like you don't have support when life gets tough, or struggle to open up to others. That can challenge your ability to make or keep relationships until you iron out the kinks. But, hey, remember, there's evidence that you can grow out of it!

I know you know how much can get in the way of your mom coming through as nurturer-in-chief (see chapter two). Still, I feel like it's important to reiterate that, indeed, shit happens. Depression or any mental health condition is not your mom's fault (though it is their responsibility to seek treatment or support for whatever they're dealing with). All moms occasionally take their hands off the maternal-sensitivity wheel to pay the damn bills or deal with life. But let the record show that your mom's behavior has consequences. Just because they didn't *mean* to mess with how you act in relationships doesn't mean they didn't do so.

THE RELATIONSHIP MOST IMPACTED BY YOUR EARLY ATTACHMENT TO YOUR MOM COULD BE . . . THE ONE WITH YOUR MOM

Like I said, there is a chance that the way you feel about yourself within your adult friendships and romantic relationships has roots in how your mom treated you as you were growing up. That is true. But, as Dr. Gillath and co-authors write in *Adult Attachment*, your early relationship with your caregivers may be more likely to influence how you relate to your *caregivers* as a grown adult than how you relate to other people.

That could mean, if your mom wasn't really there for you as a kid, you could have a relatively healthy dating life and best friends who you fully trust . . . while also feeling insecure about whether your mom cares about you. You can be secure in your friendships and love life without ever outgrowing that insecure attachment to your mom.

That's especially true if your relationship has basically stayed the same since childhood. When your mom still never asks about your interests or friends, it makes sense that you'd feel as insecure with them now as you did when you were little. Unfortunately, that's unlikely to change—unless they do. If you want to get a sense of your attachment to your mom, take the questionnaire at the end of this chapter to calculate where you stand right now.

Your mom's baggage becomes yours.

Growing up, we're basically little sociologists, observing our parents in their natural habitat. We see the way they treat us, our siblings, our other parents, extended family, random neighbors, and, of course, themselves. We also witness how they respond to conflict, challenges, good and bad news, and their own feelings.

Pharaon says we see the world through the lens of our primary caregivers until we're old enough to develop unique thoughts and opinions and identify our emotions. All of that information helps us understand the nuances of humankind and our place within it.

When our moms model healthy responses to whatever life hands them, they enable us to feel safe and calm. As a little guy, you might not know about all the problems in your mom's world. But if they're handling them like an emotionally mature champ, you go on to believe that life is generally manageable.

Of course, for unlimited reasons (see chapter two), our moms' responses *aren't* always healthy. This seems like a Them Problem, but it makes an imprint on us (just as their parents made an imprint on them). "What's not resolved in mom gets passed along to us in some form," Pharaon explains. That's because, when our caregivers don't process issues from their past, those issues can make their way into our lives in unhealthy ways, she adds.

Sometimes, those issues come in the form of a maladaptive coping mechanism. Say every time your mom was upset, she packed you in the car and headed to the mall for retail therapy. That's fun! But also, it can normalize the idea that feelings can be avoided by spending money. Is that the worst thing ever? Not exactly. However, if you adopt this response and make it your go-to way to deal with conflict, that could hinder your ability to spend time with and manage your emotions (not to mention the impact on your bank account). It's also possible you might have noticed the destruction of this maladaptive coping mechanism and taken a hard pass. Either way, it's influencing how you show up in life.

For clinical psychologist Dr. Wang, witnessing how her parents responded to racist interactions shaped how she used to assert herself. "Their gut response was to shut down and try to get out of the situation as fast as possible. They weren't fighting back, they weren't saying, 'Hey, that was racist,' or 'That was wrong,'" she explains. Instead, they "shut down and ran." While she understands why her parents responded the way they did, Dr. Wang says this shaped how she saw who she was in society because of her race. "I thought, *Was I somebody capable of taking up space? Is that allowed for somebody who lives in my body?*"

You can also pick up your mom's unresolved issues or beliefs without knowing their source. For example, if your mom was constantly body-checking in the mirror or talking trash about the way they looked, you might think it's normal to hate your physical form—or even hate on the features you inherited from your mom.

Or perhaps your mom was obsessed with cleaning and neatness. You might also find emotional solace in the perfection of an organized fridge—and inner turmoil in the face of a dusty surface. Or maybe you become a full-on clutter monster, vowing to never be like your mom.

In other words, you risk absorbing (in some way) the stuff that your mom never sorted out. You watch how your mom responds to a situation, you try to make sense of it, and then it shows up in your adult life in one way or another. "What we do with unresolved issues is endless," explains Pharaon.

Maybe their eating disorder doesn't become your eating disorder (though it could), but you might become critical, perfectionistic, or controlling at work or in relationships. If your mom yelled all the time, you might vow never to raise your voice or to avoid conflict at all costs.

We're influenced by our moms' response to life, sure. But we're also watching their response to us.

We've had much ado about the way your mom treats you as an infant and how it impacts your early attachment to them. But even as we get older, we're looking out for what gets mom's attention, what makes mom happy, what doesn't, and what that means about us.

This isn't all bad. It's useful to learn that good behavior at the grocery store makes outings a more enjoyable experience for everyone involved. Also, interrupting your mom during a phone call doesn't usually result in undivided attention. You're learning, *If I behave this way, I'm going to get a better response from my mom than if I behave this other way*, says Pharaon. That helps you develop cool things like self-control and patience. You start considering how your actions impact others. Please clap for these valuable life skills.

Alas, like other flaws in human psychology, the inclination to make your mom's actions about you can also go awry.

Perhaps your mom was always distracted when you were a kiddo, but every time you cleaned your room or helped with your siblings, mom paid attention. So what did that interaction teach you? You're most valuable when you're helping.

You also could have picked up unintended subliminal messages from your mom's depression. If being a little clown helped you get affection during her depressive episode, you might work extra hard to make a joke or be entertaining whenever possible.

Our brains pick up on negative responses too. If your mom called you dramatic or a crybaby when you came to her with tears, worries, and big feelings, you learned that hard emotions aren't welcome. With that outlook, you could start isolating from or avoiding people instead of seeking emotional support. Or you might develop a toxic level of positivity to defend against stress, anxiety, or emotions like sadness and grief. Again, how we internalize moms' feedback is endless.

Childhood adaptations aren't the end of this journey, unfortunately. Over time, the lessons we pick up as kids can become unconscious patterns or parts of our personality, explains Pharaon.

If your brain says productivity gets you attention and love, your boundaries at work might be paper-thin. You answer emails at unhinged hours, take on more work instead of delegating it, and refuse to use those sick days. Your boss probably loves you, but you're still striving to impress them (maybe for the wrong reasons?).

If it wasn't OK as a child to emote anything other than happiness, you might reflexively find the bright side. That optimistic outlook might keep the vibes high most of the time, but refusing to embrace dark feelings isn't sustainable long-term (enter the impromptu emotional outburst in line at CVS).

It's not like all of these adaptations are negative. You could have become the most hilarious person you know. Love that for you! However, when these skills become your default ways of coping in the face of adversity, they can lead you astray.

As a result, you might be paralyzed by conflict, function in a way that doesn't align with your values, or keep dating the wrong people. You might even wind up in therapy trying to figure out why the hell the same annoying stuff keeps happening to you.

Your relationship with your mom feels off.

Back in chapter one, we talked about research suggesting that most people in early adulthood consider their mom a part of their inner circle, or even one of their two closest attachment figures. But your closest or most important relationship isn't always your *healthiest.*

Anyone who has been in a terrible long-term relationship knows that you can definitely be attached to someone who doesn't treat you well. The same can be true of our attachment to our moms. "A person can play an emotionally important role in [another] person's life, even if the relationship is a conflictual one," write Dr. Gillath and colleagues in *Adult Attachment.*

Let's pause here, because this was a big epiphany for me.

For many of us, when things go wrong, we're calling mom. When things go extremely right, mom is the first or second person we tell. And when life is fine but we feel like chatting for no reason, mom is near the top of the list too.

At the same time, we don't all have healthy, happy, secure relationships with our moms (hi!). Maybe our calls are met with an indifferent, unattuned, cold, or inconsistent response. Or our moms are distracted when we're together. Our moms don't try to understand our feelings. Our moms don't show up for important moments. Our moms make everything about themselves. You probably have your own examples to add to this list.

This means many of us (again, hello!) have been out here functioning as if our "closest," "most important" relationship is warm, caring, and uplifting—when it's not.

We're staying in touch, updating them on our lives, confiding in them when it's tough out here. Yet, for reasons we can or can't put our finger on, this relationship makes us feel bad.

As far as I can tell, this data explains FOMOM (fear of missing out on mom, something I just made up). It's why we sense that we're missing the feel-good relationship everyone else seems to have with their moms. It could be why we feel less than or different from other people.

Society and our social circles reinforce the idea—whether based in truth or mass fakery—that most moms *are* a healthy, reliable source of support for young adults. Exhibit A: Your Instagram feed on Mother's Day. Exhibit B: Your college roommate adorably FaceTiming their mom twice a week. Exhibit C: Your friend with kids praising their mom's childcare abilities.

So if you continue to feel hurt, scammed, or not as good as everyone else—even as a grown person who "should be over it"—there's a reason. It's normal to want our mamas, even if they don't take good care of us.

WHAT'S YOUR ATTACHMENT STYLE TO YOUR MOM?

As I said, the relationship most likely to be impacted by your early attachment to your mom may be the one with your mom. While we might have an idea of how we show up in this relationship, having tangible data to back you up is always validating. Also, who doesn't love a personality quiz?

We've talked through the different kinds of insecure attachment styles, like anxious attachment, avoidant attachment, and disorganized attachment. But those terms don't fully capture the nuances of attachment theory.

Current attachment theory research measures attachment styles dimensionally, assessing the behavior (like hyper-independence or clinginess) and the feelings behind them. This helps researchers better understand someone's attachment style and also the motivations underlying avoidant or anxious behavior. That level of detail is extra helpful in distinguishing your specific brand of attachment in any given dynamic.

Another cool thing about attachment styles? Not only can you have a different one for every relationship; they also can change over time. So if someone proves to you that they're trustworthy, your attachment to them can become more secure.

Use this quiz to determine your attachment style with your mom.* Then read on to find out what that says about your current relationship with them.

Instructions

For each statement in the following two sections, circle the number that aligns with your feelings toward your mom right now (that last part is important for accuracy). When you're done, add up the numbers and divide them by the number of questions in that section. For this and other quizzes in the book, you will probably get a funky number with a decimal, and that's OK.

---

* Adapted from the Experiences in Close Relationships-Revised (ECR-R) adult attachment questionnaire, developed by R. Chris Fraley, Neils G. Waller, and Kelly A. Brennan, PhD, and published in 2000 in the *Journal of Personality and Social Psychology.*

Section 1: Attachment Anxiety

Attachment anxiety is characterized by "low self-worth and a fear of abandonment and rejection," according to Dr. Gillath and colleagues in *Adult Attachment*. They add that attachment anxiety can make you extra sensitive to signs someone is expressing love and rejection (again, this can be specific to your relationship with one person).

1. **I worry that my mom won't care about me as much as I care about them.**
   strongly disagree 1 2 3 4 5 6 7 strongly agree
2. **I often worry that my mom doesn't really care for me.**
   strongly disagree 1 2 3 4 5 6 7 strongly agree
3. **I'm afraid that my mom may abandon me.**
   strongly disagree 1 2 3 4 5 6 7 strongly agree

TOTAL SCORE ____ DIVIDED BY 3 = ____

Section 2: Attachment Avoidance

Attachment avoidance shows up as "discomfort with closeness, excessive self-reliance, and a lack of confidence in depending on others to meet needs for comfort and security," write Dr. Gillath and colleagues. Within an avoidantly attached relationship, you might resist seeking help, comfort, or connection with the other person.

1. **I prefer not to show my mom how I feel deep down.**
   strongly disagree 1 2 3 4 5 6 7 strongly agree

2. **I don't feel comfortable opening up to my mom.**

   strongly disagree 1 2 3 4 5 6 7 strongly agree

3. **I usually discuss my problems and concerns with my mom.**

   strongly disagree 7 6 5 4 3 2 1 strongly agree

4. **I talk things over with my mom.**

   strongly disagree 7 6 5 4 3 2 1 strongly agree

5. **I find it easy to depend on my mom.**

   strongly disagree 7 6 5 4 3 2 1 strongly agree

6. **It helps to turn to my mom in times of need.**

   strongly disagree 7 6 5 4 3 2 1 strongly agree

TOTAL SCORE ____ DIVIDED BY 6 = ____

Scoring

On the attachment style matrix that follows, use your attachment anxiety score (bottom scale) and your attachment avoidance score (left scale) to find your spot on the matrix by placing a finger on each scale number and sliding them up and across until they meet. (This message is brought to you by fifth-grade math.)

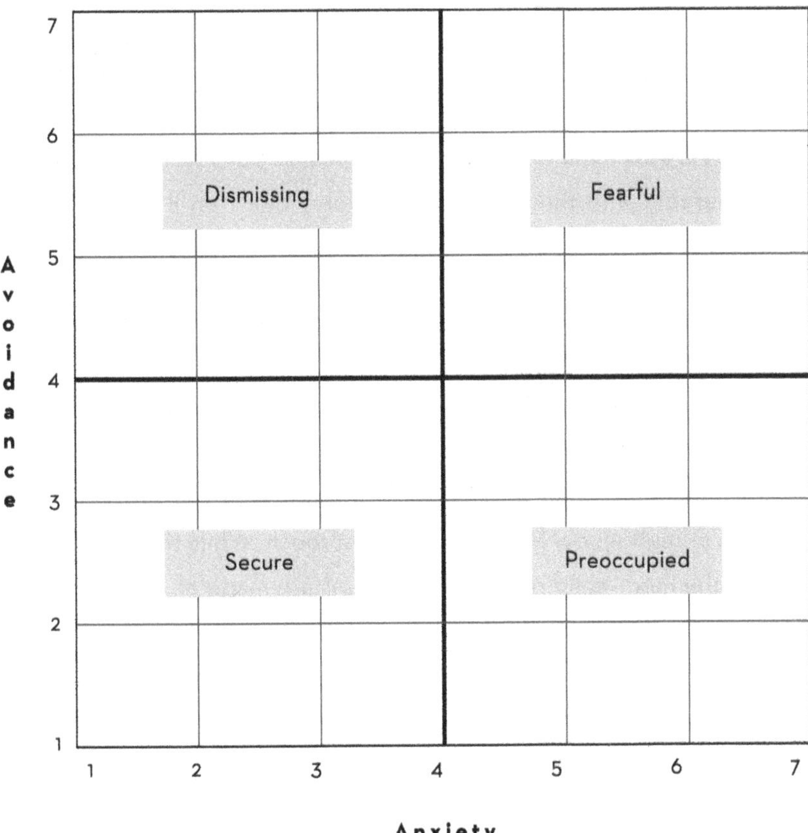

Secure: Welcome to the safety zone. If you landed in this quadrant, your relationship is relatively low in anxiety and avoidance. It's easy for you to be emotionally close with your mom, and you feel comfortable doing so. You feel cared for by your mom, and free to be yourself. You likely also feel safe depending on her. You know she'll have your back. Even if you landed on the edge of this field, chances are you're pretty secure. Still, there's always room to become closer and more securely attached.

Fearful: On the other end of the matrix lies the highly anxious and highly avoidant piece of the attachment puzzle. If you're somewhere in here, you likely avoid confiding in or depending on your mom in any way. However, the reason might be because you feel insecure and too vulnerable with them. Maybe you worry that they'll use your words against you or let you down if you ask them for help.

Dismissing: You're in the zone of, "Nah, I'm good." Landing in this quadrant means you don't like depending on your mom, you don't like your mom depending on you, and you're not worried whether or not they care about you. In the context of non-mom relationships, this might describe a dynamic with coworkers you don't get along with or high school frenemies who lost touch. While this attachment is not the mom-child relationship dreams are made of, if your mom has proven countless times that they can't be trusted, dismissing could be the safest place for you. If you found yourself here, it might indicate that you've accepted that your mom can't or won't provide closeness, intimacy, or safety. If that tracks for you, be proud of yourself.

Preoccupied: When you're low on avoidance and high on anxiety, you'll wind up here. This type of attachment to your mom can look like working hard to establish a close connection and worrying that your actions won't be reciprocated. You want a deeper, more secure, loving relationship. Still, you suspect your mom is unwilling to get close to you. It can seem like, no matter what you do, your mom doesn't care for you as much as you care for them.

CHAPTER 4

*How Unfortunate Mom Behavior Motherf*cks Us*

Now that we've got a better understanding of how moms can infiltrate our adult lives, it's time to name names. More specifically, it's time to call out the common yet problematic behaviors sometimes perpetrated by moms.

As we've established, not all moms have bad intentions. The way they were raised, the trauma they experienced, the chaos life threw at them, and the cultural norms that pressured them all contribute to the way they interact with us.

So I'd guess that, most of the time, moms who messed up didn't set out to do so. They might have truly been trying (their version of) their best or were completely unaware of the consequences of their actions. But even those who didn't set out to be the worst sometimes are.

We've mostly talked in generalities about how our moms' behavior influences the way we do life. Moms often contribute to the way we view the world. How they treat us as children can influence the health of our future relationships and instill unhelpful coping mechanisms or habits we can't shake.

While that's all validating information, there's serious power in the specifics. Anyone who's labeled their ex a gaslighter knows the sweet, sweet relief of putting a name to a painful experience. That's what we'll be doing here: classifying the specific ways your mom went wrong and how they could be impacting your life now.

Naming a behavior can do a thing mental health pros call externalizing, or redefining a difficulty as an external problem rather than an internal one.

When you're able to name a thing you experienced, it exists outside of you. If you used to think, *Well, I was a really annoying kid* or *I should have just handled my mom differently*, calling out the messed-up way they treated you can stop you from blaming yourself.

To be clear, this chapter is not about to diagnose your mom or testify on your behalf in a court of law. But it could cosign what you've been through and the repercussions. Categorizing your experiences with your mom as unhealthy, emotionally immature, or abusive behavior can help you make sense of your feelings about them. The thing that made you feel bad *was* bad.

You weren't being needy or blowing things out of proportion, you were experiencing something universally shitty. Maybe you didn't have the words to explain it before, but now you do. In times of doubt or self-blame, you can say, "This is what happened to me." You're right to be hurt, upset, or traumatized. That thing *was* a messed-up thing!

You can call your friends and say, "Turns out, I was being parentified!" You can look back on some of the most hurtful experiences with your mom and call that shit what it is: *I see you, emotional manipulation!* or *Damn, that was child abuse.*

When you name the way someone treated you, it can be easier to process what happened, how it made you feel, and what you want to do about it.

It also helps you feel less alone. If there's a term for what your mom did (or is doing) to you, then you can't be the only one to have experienced it. This behavior happens so often that it has a *name.* In a world where we assume everyone has a perfect relationship with their moms, having vocab for our situation makes us feel more normal.

With all of that in mind, we'll be chugging through different categories of maltreatment. Some of these are actual psychological or legal terms and some are names I made up to classify types of behavior that I've grouped together for easier processing. In both cases, we'll talk through some of the ways these harmful actions (or inaction) might be influencing your life today, including your relationship with your mom right now.

But first, a sensitivity warning: The rest of this chapter will describe some forms of child abuse, sexual abuse, and abusive relationships in general. Please proceed with caution and ensure you have the appropriate coping tools in place to help you spend time with and manage your emotions. If you want to skip the rest of this chapter, that's fine too. I'll see you in part two on page 89.

WHEN NAMING NAMES SETS YOU BACK

While identifying problematic behaviors can help us move forward, it can also keep some people stuck. Understandably, not everyone responds to labels like "emotional abuse" or "negligence" in constructive ways, says Minaa B., therapist and author of *Owning Our Struggles.*

For example, maybe "abuse" feels like too strong of a word, even if your mom's behavior meets the criteria for it. If your idea of what a label means keeps you from believing your experience, that's not helpful.

It's also not great if the technical term for your mom's treatment makes you feel like damaged goods, irrevocably messed up.

When that kind of thing happens, Minaa B. suggests throwing the name out altogether. You don't need to categorize it to address the behavior it describes.

Instead, think about the behavior itself. What was your experience? How did it make you feel? Does it align with what you'd call a healthy relationship? That little thought exercise can help you acknowledge what happened without those unhelpful side effects.

ABUSE

For all the reasons we talked about in chapter two, sometimes moms abuse their children. There are different types of abuse—physical, sexual, and emotional—but these categories often overlap. Your mom could slap you for getting bad grades, making you feel ashamed (emotional abuse) and inflicting physical pain (physical abuse) at the same time.

If this happens when you're under the age of eighteen, it's called child abuse. Child abuse is illegal, and we'll definitely be getting into that. Before we do, though, you might need to hear that adults can experience abusive behavior from their moms too.

Say your mom has consistently criticized your weight since you were little. Back then, it consisted of calling you harsh nicknames. These days, it might look like judgmental comments when you're eating together or intentionally gifting you clothes that are too small. While it's still emotional abuse, once you're over eighteen, it's no longer child abuse.

If you suspect you experienced or are experiencing abuse but have a hard time acknowledging that, stigma could be to blame. Minaa B.

reminds us that society has a pretty stereotyped view of what it means to be "an abuser"—that they're damaged, dangerous people who can't be rehabilitated. This makes the label of "abuse" or "abuser" hard to apply to the person who raised you. It taints the perception of who your mom is and who you are.

You might think, *What does it say about me if I came from an abusive home or had an abusive childhood?* You might worry that it would change how you or others see you and your childhood.

Abusive behavior can also be tough to spot if you don't know any different or it's normalized in the culture in which you grew up, Minaa B. explains.

Believing yourself makes the abuse real, which hurts. So instead of facing it, we sometimes try to make the behavior make sense by renaming what happened, blaming it on external circumstances, blaming ourselves, or even pretending it didn't happen. Explaining it away helps us cope when the people meant to protect and love us harm us, says Minaa B.

When we were kids, those protective measures kept us safe and attached to the people we rely on. As adults, who don't need that protection, avoiding the truth can keep us stuck in old patterns with our moms.

With all that in mind, let's talk about what child abuse is, according to the federal and state laws that outline it and the mental health pros who've studied it.

Definitions of abuse vary from state to state, but federal law—specifically the Child Abuse Prevention and Treatment Act (CAPTA)—defines child abuse as "any recent act or failure to act on the part of a parent or caretaker which results in death, serious physical or emotional harm, sexual abuse or exploitation" of, or "an act or failure to act which presents an imminent risk of serious harm" to, a person under the age of eighteen.

OK, yes, this is kind of a broad, vague criterion, but here's how Minaa B. explains child abuse in the most basic terms: Abuse is a pattern of intentional harm or mistreatment that affects you physically, mentally, or emotionally.

Often, the person who is abusing you will encourage you not to tell anyone. They may threaten you or make you feel as if they may harm you more if you say something.

Physical Child Abuse

Physical child abuse happens any time a parent injures a kid on purpose. Most states also say that creating circumstances that threaten a kid's life or health counts too.

That means physical child abuse could be things like hitting or kicking, and also driving you to soccer practice after several glasses of wine, per the definition laid out in CAPTA. Letting someone else physically harm you also falls in this category of abuse.

As we discussed, if you're raised in a family that is down with spanking or other forms of physical punishment, it can be hard to reconcile that with a label like child abuse.

Sexual Child Abuse

Sexual abuse is another physical form of illegal child mistreatment. Here's how CAPTA defines it: "the employment, use, persuasion, inducement, enticement, or coercion of any child to engage in, or assist any other person to engage in, any sexually explicit conduct or simulation of such conduct for the purpose of producing a visual depiction of such conduct; or the rape, and in cases of caretaker or interfamilial relationships, statutory rape, molestation, prostitution, or other forms of sexual exploitation of children, or incest with children."

Touching or engaging you sexually, letting others do it, and making you pretend to do something sexual are sexual abuse. Any kind of sexual interaction involving a child is sexual abuse.

Emotional Child Abuse

Because there are no physical interactions between the abuser and child—and thus no marks—emotional child abuse can be harder to identify. That said, emotional abuse is when someone repeatedly manipulates, threatens, or belittles you, often in hopes of a desired outcome, says Minaa B.

Legally speaking, more than half of states define emotional abuse as "injury to the psychological capacity or emotional stability of the child as evidenced by an observable or substantial change in behavior, emotional response, or cognition," and harm indicated by "anxiety, depression, withdrawal, or aggressive behavior," per the Child Welfare Information Gateway (CWIG).

That means, depending on where you live, you might need to show changes in your behavior or even receive a legit mental health diagnosis as a kid for the treatment to be emotional abuse in the eyes of the law. Honestly, that's a high bar.

While there's no list of actions that define emotionally abusive behavior in every state, emotional abuse could look like:

* Yelling in a scary or threatening way
* Calling you names
* Isolating you from other people
* Ignoring you on purpose as punishment (the silent treatment)
* Sharing inappropriate information with you
* Embarrassing you in front of others on purpose

* Blaming you for things that are not your fault or are out of your control
* Exposing you to harmful relationships or substance use
* Threatening you, your stuff, or people and pets you love
* Bullying you
* Restricting your access to basic needs, like bathing, food, or a place to sleep

All of these behaviors make a child feel unsafe, unloved, and unimportant, and can have massive emotional repercussions.

Signs It Happened to You

There are a ton of nuanced ways being abused can show up in your life now. It would be impossible to cover them all here, but Minaa B. says these are some common ways childhood abuse can impact you as an adult:

* Difficulty having hard conversations without fear of backlash or being punished
* Joking around during serious moments to ease tension, even when it's not necessary
* Avoiding emotional expression, vulnerability, or talking about your feelings with others
* Feeling numb in platonic and romantic relationships
* Feeling insecure in any kind of relationship
* Being clingy or avoidant (or both) in relationships
* Needing constant reassurance that people like you
* Suspecting that you're not good enough
* Distrusting others
* Guarding yourself in both platonic and romantic relationships

* Repeating the same harmful behavior as your mom (or other caregivers), like physical violence, yelling, and emotional manipulation
* Consistently sacrificing your needs and wants for others (see also: people pleasing)
* Being hyper-independent, avoiding reliance on anyone for anything

Understandably, your mom's abusive behavior can also impact your relationship with her. Here's how that often looks, according to Minaa B.:

* Feeling psychologically unsafe with your mom
* Avoiding emotional closeness by not confiding in her, telling her about certain milestones, sharing things you think she'll ridicule you for, or asking for help
* Keeping secrets from her to protect yourself or prevent conflict
* Having mixed emotions about her, like not feeling close to her while feeling guilty that you don't have a better relationship
* Feeling grief or like you're mourning a relationship you never had

IF IT'S NOT ILLEGAL, IS IT ABUSE?

During a session with my therapist, I explained (again) why I still called my mom every other week despite consistently feeling like shit afterward.

I told her that my mom never beat me up or forgot to feed me. Putting up boundaries felt disproportionate to the problem . . . a problem I'd spent almost all of my therapy sessions for the previous three years addressing. I reasoned that distancing yourself from your mom requires a good excuse. For me, it felt like an overreaction.

Then my therapist said, "So, she never did anything illegal. Does that mean it wasn't abuse?"

To that, I now say, *Touché, milady.*

As Minaa B. said, *any* pattern of intentional physical, mental, or emotional mistreatment is abusive. So, does your mom's behavior have to be illegal to be abusive? Nope. It does not. (And for what it's worth, your mom's actions don't have to have been abusive to have been harmful.)

Welcome to the very gray area between illegal child abuse and the classic characteristics of a dysfunctional family.

To make sense of this space, I bring you the relationship spectrum, created by LoveIsRespect.org (part of the National Domestic Violence Hotline). This tool illustrates the characteristics of healthy relationships, abusive relationships, and a secret third option, "unhealthy" relationships.

In healthy relationships, both parties communicate with each other, treat each other with respect and trust, prioritize honesty (within reason), give each other space, give input on decisions, respect boundaries, and have access to financial means. As far as I can tell, those traits hold up for relationships between kids and their moms too.

On the other end of the healthy-relationship spectrum is abusive behavior, like making threats or saying hurtful things; dismissing your thoughts, feelings, decisions, and opinions; accusing you of doing things you're not; and (naturally) denying that they're doing anything wrong.

Last, we have the category most of us here likely fall into: unhealthy relationships. With this type, behaviors may not be abusive, but they still cause harm.

Signs of an unhealthy relationship include fighting when issues arise or not talking about them at all. Also in this category: being inconsiderate of the other person's feelings, not believing the other person will do what they say, overruling the other person's opinions, and restricting how much time the other person spends away.

If you can relate, your mom might have yelled at you instead of trying to understand you. She could have been unpredictable, saying one thing but doing another.

A lot of the behaviors described in the rest of this chapter can also be forms of abuse. Or they might "just" be symptoms of an unhealthy relationship. The most important part is that these behaviors happened and they hurt you—however you choose to label them.

CONTROLLING AND TROLLING

One of the coolest parts about a healthy relationship with your mom is the freedom to be yourself. You can be weird, outgoing, quiet, introverted, and very into anime and reptiles—or fashion and highbrow literature. You can move across the country and date someone totally different than your family. And you can do all of that without your mom judging you (or, at least, outwardly doing so). They don't attempt to change you in some way.

But not all moms are down to let their kids be who they are. Maybe your mom micromanages you or makes deliberately offensive remarks about you, making you second-guess your choices. These behaviors prioritize their expectations over your need to be an autonomous person. Whether your mom's actions match one or more of the following examples, or take another form, the main objective of controlling and trolling behavior is to manipulate you into doing and being something else.

Emotional Manipulation

FYI, most of the stuff in this chapter is a form of emotional manipulation, which is any behavior that attempts to control you via your emotions. Said emotions can include fear, guilt, obligation, insecurity, shame, or any other feeling they can exploit to influence you.

Because we're all sort of walking around with an invisible umbilical cord (as Minaa B. puts it), a guilt trip or judgmental comment from your mom can be more intense than it would be from anyone else. The fear of hurting your mom's feelings, jeopardizing her love for you, or making her unhappy is powerful. When your mom makes your behavior about her, you might decide that her contentment is more important than your safety or sanity.

Behavioral Control

As kids, we need boundaries—often in the form of rules—to feel safe and learn what behaviors are helpful (studying) and which are less so (playing video games till 4 AM). Those boundaries are forms of behavioral control, which is a generally OK thing, even a necessary one—as long as those controls lessen over time.

If your mom enforces rules that feel overly protective or out of step with your development—like patrolling the kind of music you can listen to as a teenager or where you work as an adult—she might be exerting too much behavioral control over you. Over time, an inappropriate level of behavioral control can keep you from thinking critically or inhibit self-discovery.

Psychological Control

Unlike behavioral control, which aims to dictate your actions, psychological control attempts to manage your thoughts, feelings, and opinions. That's quite dangerous, actually. It shows you that you're not free to be yourself, find your own way, or be anything other than what your mom wants.

Psychological control can come in the form of critiquing how you express yourself or pretending not to hear you talk about your interests. It can also show up as scoffing or an epic eyeroll when you give your opinion or (God forbid) feedback about how your mom's actions make you feel.

Criticism

In the context of parenting, this term describes "negative statements designed to stop or change children's undesirable behavior or communicate displeasure with the child," per a study in the *Journal of Pediatric Health Care*.

As any parent will tell you, critiquing a kid's behavior is part of teaching them how to be a person. When moms tell us to take a bath or stop throwing food on the floor, we're learning important things.

Taken too far, though, these critiques can mess with our self-esteem, hurt our feelings, and make us act out. If your mom calls you names, makes fun of how you look or act, critiques your body, belittles your interests or work, or comes at you in an otherwise rude, judgey, inconsiderate way, you learn things like your preferences don't matter and your ideas are stupid.

Physical Threats

Another way caregivers can control what we do, say, or think is by threatening to hurt us or come for the people, pets, and things we love. Even if your mom never does it, saying she will makes us feel unsafe. She could even use language like "I hope your dog runs away and never comes back." She's not saying she'll make it happen, but the fact that she wants a thing you care about to disappear is terrifying.

Conditional Love and Attention

You've probably heard of unconditional love. It's the kind of affection and care we should get from our parents: paying attention to us, cheering us on, snuggling us, encouraging us, and meeting our needs without expectations of reciprocity.

It doesn't matter if we fail a class, get kicked off a team, embrace goth culture, or choose a career path they wouldn't. We're still entitled (yeah, entitled!) to their love, attention, and understanding.

Conditional love is the opposite of that. It's when your caregiver retaliates after you do something that displeases them, even if that's just being yourself. They withhold love and affection, verbally tear you to shreds, or just drop a sarcastic, "Oh, that's interesting." Their love for you (or at least the expression of it) is only given if you meet their benchmarks.

Of course, that assumes said caregiver shows you love the rest of the time. For some, that's not the case. If feeling loved and cared for by your mom isn't the norm, and her affection appears only when you do something she likes, that's conditional love too.

Signs It Happened to You

In a perfect world, our caregivers are the ones who embrace who we are even before we know who that is. When they don't, it changes how we show up in the world and how we see ourselves. Minaa B. notes that if you've been controlled and trolled in childhood and/or beyond, those repercussions can show up in the following ways:

* Feeling developmentally stunted
* Having a hard time with critical thinking
* Struggling to build social connections (especially if your mom isolated you)
* Feeling unsure of what you want for yourself outside of what your mom wants
* Rebelling against your mom or family in big, sometimes dangerous ways
* Second-guessing or doubting yourself more often than not
* Feeling like you're not good enough
* Feeling like a fraud despite being very qualified and accomplished (see: impostor syndrome)
* Hyperfixating on parts of your body you want to change
* Feeling like everyone is judging or critiquing you in social situations (social anxiety)

A lot of these controlling and trolling behaviors betray trust and can make us feel unsafe around the person we're taught should have our back more than anyone else. That's why the fallout is often similar to that of abusive behaviors, says Minaa B. You might avoid closeness with your mom, keep big parts of your life private from her, and feel mixed emotions about all that.

YOU DO YOU-ING

As we discussed earlier, our craving for mom-based attention and affection doesn't go away as we age. That's why the kind of behavior that makes you feel like you're on your own can hurt even as an adult.

When our moms leave us hanging physically or emotionally, they're telling us they're out—"You do you, my child." Whether this behavior is a result of your mom's maladaptive coping mechanisms or some rough circumstances, she's putting her trauma, emotional immaturity, or life before your well-being. Here's what that can look like.

Physical Neglect

Though definitions can vary, child neglect per the CWIG is a type of physical abuse in which your caregivers don't provide food, shelter, medical care, or clothing to the point that it becomes dangerous. If you experienced periods without access to meals, clean clothes, or a place to sleep, you likely experienced neglect in its most severe form.

As you know, abusive behaviors aren't always illegal—and their legality doesn't make them any less harmful. That's true for neglect as well. For example, if you never felt prepared for school because no one was around to help you with your homework, or your caregiver assumed you were good just figuring it out on your own, that could also be neglect.

This kind of you-do-you behavior might have left you feeling alone as a kid or young adult. You might have had to figure basic things out on your own, like how to get yourself to school, cook, do your hair, or wash your clothes. Maybe you didn't figure those things out till much later in life.

Abandonment

Sometimes caregivers leave. Whether it's forever or for a period when you really needed them, abandonment means they left you. If this sounds like neglect, that's because abandonment can be a form of it.

Maybe your mom left you at home alone for long periods of time. Or maybe she left you in a car whenever she went into a store. Whatever it looked like, she abdicated her parental responsibilities.

As an adult, you can still be abandoned. Though it's not against the law for a parent to cut off contact with you, doing so can be a form of abandonment. Or let's say you approach your mom about a conflict or a problem you want to work through with her. If she responds by not responding, completely ghosting you, it's safe to say she's abandoning you. And given how much power parents can still hold in their relationship with their adult kids, that abandonment can be painful.

Emotional Neglect

It's not always easy for a parent to manage a kid's feelings along with all the other stuff happening in their life. Even the best parents sometimes get overwhelmed. But when a parent consistently disregards, ignores, or dismisses their child's emotional needs or belittles them for having feelings, that's emotional neglect.

Even if you have clothes, a fridge full of food, and someone to take you to and from Little League, that's not enough to thrive, unfortunately. If your mom isn't checking in on you, creating a safe space to share your feelings, or validating your emotions, you quickly learn that emotions don't matter (or, at least, yours don't). You might also decide that feeling things annoys people, especially your mom. That can make you feel incredibly alone or even unsafe around her.

One of Foxy's go-to catchphrases is, "It's your life." It's hard to remember when she started dropping this line on me, but if I had to make an educated guess, I'd say middle school.

She often presented it when I shared personal things about myself, including my feelings, my plans for the future, or my opinion on anything—especially if she didn't understand or agree with it. This continued through college and beyond.

Instead of engaging in a conversation to learn more about who I am, my motivations, or my taste in TJ Maxx offerings, she'd say, "It's your life," throwing my bid for connection and visibility back at me. The subtext I picked up was *I don't care.*

While emotional neglect makes a big impression on us as kids, your mom can continue to be emotionally neglectful as you get older. She might forget to ask how you're doing, sticking to surface-level questions like "How's work?" and "How's your partner?" But she skims over how you're *really* doing.

Signs It Happened to You

Minaa B. says that symptoms of neglect and abandonment are often the same as for any other emotionally abusive behavior. You might avoid vulnerability, conflict, confrontation, and trusting others. In relationships, platonic or not, you might feel insecure or numb. You might keep things surface level to protect yourself and get the ick when someone leans on you for support.

Plus, Dr. Kathryn Humphreys of Vanderbilt University says that, if you don't receive attuned care starting in early childhood, it can dysregulate your sense of what's normal in relationships. Over time, that can make you less likely to find friends and partners who value you, she explains.

Your relationship with your mom takes a hit too. Even as an adult, you probably feel unsafe with her, avoid emotional closeness, and feel bad about your relationship looking different than your friends' relationships with their moms.

DUMPING

You might not always realize when you're a victim of underage emotional labor. When parents employ us as sounding boards, therapists, or close friends, it can feel kinda nice—until it doesn't.

Though taking on your mom's drama can happen (and sucks) at any age, it can be particularly damaging for kids. When we're young, it can feel empowering for us to step up to the plate. The reflex to help when our moms need an ear or a hand also comes naturally. Moms' safety and security determine our safety and security, and we benefit when we maintain it. Here we are to save the fucking day.

But things can go wrong when our moms put this kind of undue pressure on us. Here are the most common ways our moms dump on us and what that looks like.

Parentifying

Parentification happens when a parent makes their needs your problem. More specifically, it's "a parent–child dynamic in which children assume caregiving responsibilities while parents fail to support and reciprocate children's roles," according to researchers who study this stuff for a living.

It could look like having to wake your mom up to take you to school and remind her of doctor's appointments or parent–teacher conferences so she doesn't miss them. It might also show up in less obvious ways, like being asked to discipline your siblings or put in the middle of conflicts with other adults.

Like many of the behaviors in this chapter, parentification exists along a spectrum. On one end, you could have something like helping one parent care for another during a health emergency (like a sixteen-year-old making a meal or driving their parent to a doctor's appointment). On the other end, you might have been paying bills, managing schedules, doing most of the chores, and becoming the primary caregiver for siblings or even a parent. Some research suggests that the younger you are when this starts, the more severe the psychological impact.

Enmeshment

Like parentifying, enmeshment puts too much responsibility on the person with the least power in a family (see: the child). With enmeshment, though, the load you're carrying is mostly emotional.

The American Psychological Association describes enmeshment as "a condition in which two or more people, typically family members, are involved in each other's activities and personal relationships to an excessive degree, thus limiting or precluding healthy interaction and compromising individual autonomy and identity."

If you're enmeshed with your mom, she might be overly intrusive about what's happening in your personal life; feel entitled to access you whenever she wants; and/or expect you to have the same thoughts, values, feelings, and opinions as she does. If you don't, she might guilt or shame you into hiding your true self. She could also get extra emotional in hopes that you'll feel bad for her (emotional manipulation at its finest!).

Enmeshment can also happen if your mom unloads her personal struggles onto you. Just a heads-up: When you were a kid, it was never OK for your mom to vent to you about age-inappropriate issues in her romantic relationships (especially with your other parent), friendships, or with family members, or about adult stressors at work. She shouldn't expect you to be there for her like a therapist, close friend, or partner.

While it makes sense for conversations to mature as you age, children don't have the bandwidth or skills to help their moms navigate the adult world. Tasking them with this job violates the healthy boundaries between a parent and child, blurring the kid's role in the relationship.

When this kind of behavior is consistent, it becomes hard to separate your emotions from your mom's. When she's freaked out, you're freaked out. When she's going through a rough patch at work or with your other parent, you feel on edge and anxious too. Her struggles become yours, and your ability to be a kid or grow into your own person leaves the chat.

Signs It Happened to You

While parentification and enmeshment both put tons of inappropriate pressure on you, Minaa B. finds that the consequences can vary.

Parentification

* Taking on a caretaker role in your adult relationships with friends or partners
* Chronic people pleasing or having a hard time saying no
* Feeling like you need to solve everyone's problems or rescue people you're close with
* Consistently allowing others to push past your boundaries

* Not giving friends, family, or partners a chance to support you
* Feeling like you have to have all the answers
* Avoiding closeness because you're worried others will want too much from you

Enmeshment

In Minaa B.'s experience, people who were enmeshed with their mom at an early age might also deal with the just-listed symptoms of parentification. They likely also have challenges similar to those who were controlled by their moms (see "Controlling and Trolling" from earlier). Here's a reminder of what that could look like:

* Feeling developmentally stunted
* Having a hard time with critical thinking
* Struggling to build social connections (especially if your mom isolated you)
* Feeling unsure of what you want for yourself outside of what your mom wants from you
* Rebelling against your mom or family in big, sometimes dangerous ways
* Second-guessing yourself more often than not
* Doubting or not trusting yourself

Like the other categories of behavior we talked about, dumping can make adult you feel uneasy and on guard around your mom. You might find yourself stuck in those old parentified or enmeshed patterns, putting your mom's wants, needs, and feelings ahead of your own. You might feel like you owe her because she paid for your schooling or kept you fed and clothed. You also might worry she's still incapable of caring for herself or being independent. Patterns can be hard to break.

WHAT'S FORGIVABLE AND WHAT ISN'T

Your mom might have done some bad things, but that doesn't mean she is necessarily irredeemable. There are plenty of situations where a mom's circumstances or maturity level could have made it extremely challenging to be there for you as a child, despite wanting to do so. And just like you, she's not the same person she was fifteen, twenty, or thirty years ago, says Minaa B.

Obviously, I would never tell you to forgive and forget your experience. I don't think any mental health professional would either. Still, dismissing your mom as a lost cause because of her past actions, especially if she's changed since (or expressed a desire to change), isn't always the move. Ultimately, you get to choose what's best for your unique situation.

SO, WHAT NOW?

Sitting with all this can bring up mental and emotional chatter. Reading examples of harmful behavior that you relate to might piss you off. You might forget about all the compassion and empathy we discussed a couple of chapters ago. That's fine! Or you might feel defensive of your mom, given whatever she's been through. That's equally acceptable.

Having compassion for our moms in all their dysfunctional glory is highly recommended by me and actual mental health professionals. Still, there's no denying their hurtful behavior fucks us up. Two facts can be true at the same time.

Minaa B. backs me up on this. You can have empathy for all the factors behind your mom's hurtful behavior, but ignoring the pain she caused is abandoning yourself. "There has to be a line that gets drawn between *I can have compassion for you, but I still have to have compassion for myself*," says Minaa B.

Another pitfall of rehashing these issues with your mom is getting caught up in blame. "I think if we are just constantly saying, *I'm this way because of my mom, and that's where the sentence ends*, that's problematic," says Vienna Pharaon, therapist and author of *The Origins of You*. "Blaming someone else does not move us forward at all. It doesn't help us."

Pharaon suggests reframing the blame as acknowledgment. You can say, *Here's what I remember. This was my experience,* she explains. From there, you can decide what you want to do about it.

And that's what we'll do in part two.

How to Heal Your Shit and Keep It That Way

CHAPTER 5

What Is Healing and How Do I Get Some?

At this point, you know why moms can take up so much of our mental space. You know that their circumstances can sometimes make being a caregiver extra challenging and even lead to harmful parenting. You also know that blaming or making excuses for your mom won't help you move forward.

If you feel hopeless, overwhelmed, and bummed that things went the way they did, I get it! The last couple of chapters were heavy and might have surfaced emotions and memories you wouldn't choose to hang out with.

But now that those big, mom-related emotions are here, we might as well use them. For better or worse, your feelings about this relationship (and its origin story) play a massive part in what comes next, or what some might call your *healing journey*.

Those italics are meant to imply a little side eye because "healing" and "journey" feel cringe to me, especially when used together. Still, I'm not sure there's a better way to describe what's about to happen here in part two.

CAN SOMEONE PLEASE EXPLAIN WHAT HEALING MEANS?

I'm sorry to report that there is no official definition of healing in an emotional context. That said, I asked a few mental health pros how they would describe it, and here's what I learned.

Emotional healing isn't that different from physical healing. The goal is to overcome your pain and go from feeling broken to feeling whole—from feeling dysfunctional to feeling functional.

Like with a physical injury, healing doesn't mean you'll go back to how you were before the painful thing happened (or how you would have been if it never did). Instead, you might learn to live with the scar tissue or modify how you do certain activities. But eventually, you shift from just getting by to living how you want.

My takeaway is this: Emotional healing is a process in which you acknowledge something that hurts, care for it, and adjust how you live to account for the pain. When you heal, you learn to deal with what happened without letting it rule you.

Could healing be described as a ~journey~? Sure. You're definitely going somewhere new. But the route isn't logical and there isn't an endpoint—especially when it comes to mom stuff.

When the thing that messed you up is a figure as omnipresent as The Mother, you may feel triggered, face setbacks, and need to find new ways to manage those triggers and setbacks for as long as you both shall live.

Also, healing isn't a process that applies just to you and your feelings about your mom. You can also heal the relationship *with* your mom, explains grief researcher Robert A. Neimeyer, PhD, author of *Living Beyond Loss: Questions and Answers about Grief and Bereavement* and director of the Portland Institute for Loss.

Like with your own healing, working on your relationship with your mom isn't about teleporting to a time when you two were cool or pretending everything is fine. The point is to confront the issues, repair what you can, and adapt to the way things stand.

This is not to say we should all be out here trying to make up with our moms. For some, that's not possible or productive. But for others, this process can help them shift expectations and find a more realistic sense of hope for future interactions (more on that soon).

HOW DOES THAT EVEN WORK?

Let me formally welcome you to the doing phase of the emotional healing process. Over the next several chapters, I'll explain what it takes to work through the fallout of your relationship with your mom and keep her toxic drama from ruining your life.

I really wish I had a PDF for you to follow, with simple, step-by-step instructions that can quickly spin a shitty relationship with your mom into pure gold. But alas, after months of reporting and decades of experience, I can confidently say that it doesn't work like that.

Here's what I've learned: The first step in the healing process is acknowledgment, or seeing a situation for what it is (what all of part one was about). Then comes grief. Now that you can see your mom's behavior in high definition, all the things she took from you or will never provide become clearer. Those are losses, and we have to spend time with them to work through your emotions and reach the third step, acceptance. Acceptance is the part of the process when you live your life in accordance with your current reality.

Sounds glorious, and it is, but unfortunately, that's not the end. Even when your grief is in full swing, or after you've finally achieved acceptance, you'll still need to manage interactions with people (Family! Friends! Your mother!) who don't understand your feelings or believe there's a problem.

Now, let me explain how these steps work together to get the job done.

Acknowledgment

This alone can be a struggle. We make excuses for our moms or come up with storylines to soften the harsh treatment we experience. It's easier—at least in the short term—to exist in a world where your mom is just misunderstood or shows her love in ways that don't always feel like love. Maybe you tell yourself that once the perfect circumstances align, your mom will become who you want her to be.

But to truly make peace with the way your mom is, you have to see her actions for what they are: unfair, hurtful, or even abusive. Acknowledging what you've experienced, looking it right in the face, and saying, *Yep, that's terrible,* is how you get started.

Grief

While acknowledging that the dynamic with your mom is really challenging, clearing that hurdle isn't enough to heal. Instead, you'll also need to sit with what the relationship will never be and the ways it failed you. That's how you reach real, lasting acceptance.

In chapter four, we talked through some of the common ways caregivers can behave badly and the consequences of those actions. What all of those harmful behaviors have in common is that they took something from you: your innocence, confidence, freedom, individuality, or safety. I could go on, and I will.

For now, though, know that a dysfunctional relationship with your mom means experiencing loss.

Let me back up a second to properly reintroduce you to the concept of loss. You're familiar with the "I'm sorry for your" kind. But loss also happens when your circumstances shift, the way you see something or someone changes, or an experience makes it impossible to revert to how things were before, writes Darcy L. Harris, PhD, in *Non-Death Loss and Grief: Context and Clinical Implications.* Anytime you can't undo, unsee, or unknow what you've been through, that's loss.

When something shatters our assumptions about how the world should work, our brains have to reconfigure our reality, Dr. Harris writes with Howard Winokuer, PhD, LPC, in *Principles and Practice of Grief Counseling, 3rd Edition*. That process can feel deeply unsafe, even if that isn't immediately obvious to you.

This is where grief comes in. Grief is the process of "adapting to a world that is different than the one we thought we were living in or *should* be living in," explains Dr. Neimeyer. By grieving, you start to rebuild your reality without the thing you lost (or never had).

Acceptance

Once you have a grasp on what went down and your emotional response to it, you can decide what to do next. That's acceptance, baby. I don't want to fangirl too hard here, but acceptance could be the key to getting over your mom drama. It's the endgame of healing. With a stronger sense of agency, you're empowered to do what's best for you. Making moves that align with your interests could literally change your life.

Boundaries

Acknowledging, grieving, and accepting aren't easy, and the work can be interrupted by people in your life who don't get what you're dealing with or don't like how you're responding to it. Those outside influences can have you second-guessing yourself or feeling like you're better off submitting to the status quo. So, creating boundaries is a nonnegotiable here too. You might set limits with yourself, your mom, or the people in your life who get in the way of your grieving process (whether they mean to or not).

THE TRACK TO HEALING

Basically, this healing journey looks like running a marathon on a track.

Acknowledgment is what kicks off the process (like the starter pistol at a track meet). To get going, you have to acknowledge that there's a problem. Your mom isn't who you want her to be, she does things that make you feel bad about yourself, and this relationship isn't working for you. Once you see that, you're off!

Then comes the grief. In this long-distance-race analogy, grief is the running. It's the work you do to reach acceptance.

Seeing your relationship with your mom for what it is means grieving what it's not. You might also need to grieve all the ways your mom let you down or how your life might be different if this relationship were healthier. That's painful, and it takes conscious effort to get through. When you push through it, though, you reach acceptance.

Acceptance is the finish line, and it's also a marker of progress (hence the track). Once you process the losses and all the emotions they bring up, you've finished a lap. You accept your mom and your relationship with them as it stands. You don't hold out hope that something will change.

But I think it's fair to assume that, most of the time, people struggling to heal from their dynamic with their mom don't have one single aspect of that relationship they need to accept. So you'll likely find yourself making laps forever. While running in circles doesn't feel great, all of that work adds up to meaningful progress.

Also, as anyone who's been through this will tell you, the longer you do it, the easier it gets. The time between grief and acceptance gets faster. And fending off haters, the unhelpfully ambivalent, or your mom's chaos becomes quick work with practice.

You may never feel amazing about your relationship with your mom, but you will be OK.

CHAPTER 6

Why Your Mom May Never Change...

When I was eight or nine, I was playing outside with my friend—let's call her Megan—when her mom came out to say Megan had to go in for the evening. As Mrs. Megan's mom crashed our party, I noticed that she played with Megan's hair and wrapped her arms around her. I walked my smelly kid self home and thought about how nice that kind of mom attention looked. I didn't really know how to classify unsolicited physical affection, but I knew I wanted some.

I kicked my shoes off in the mudroom and asked Foxy straight up, "Why don't you baby me anymore?"

It was an uncharacteristically bold move for me. It was also a genuine question. Was I missing something? Why wasn't my hair being played with? Where were my impromptu public cuddles? Why was I the one being booted out of a friend's place at dinnertime instead of the one being called in?

Foxy looked at me blankly and said, "You want me to treat you like a *baby*?"

I mean, solid burn. She had me there. Still, I wasn't a grown man with a diaper-wearing fetish (no judgment); I was a third-grader trying to get loved up and treated like the child I was. You know, *mothered*, so to speak.

As I tried to explain this, Foxy scoffed and said, "Oh, so you want a smother mother." I knew what she meant. It was a term she used for moms who seemed overly nurturing or accommodating. I felt embarrassed for wanting that, so I never brought it up again.

To make this relationship make sense, I came up with explanations for the way she treated me. She's just extremely outgoing! Sometimes that meant leaving me alone in the toilet paper aisle of Walmart while she made friends with someone working in electronics. Dementia runs in my family, so perhaps that's why she can't remember the names of friends I made after 2004, or what my long-term partner's parents look like.

Sure, she could recall the details of her gym friends' lives and everything she did for the past week (she usually spent fifteen minutes of our twenty-minute phone calls recapping it). But I assumed for a long time that there must be some medical explanation as to why her brain doesn't have space for me. To my knowledge, there isn't one.

Instead of acknowledging that these were all side effects of our (often unhealthy) dynamic, I held out hope for decades that Foxy could become the person I needed or wanted her to be—but it was up to me to change her. I just had to be vigilant.

When I was in elementary school, I asked her to put notes in my lunchbox and (in her words) treat me like a baby. When I was in high school, I often volunteered to do her hair and makeup, a "bonding" moment she tolerated. Well into my twenties, I made disturbingly detailed Christmas lists. That way, I wouldn't be disappointed when Foxy gifted me more physical evidence that she didn't know much about who I was or what I liked.

I'd also highlight the fun parts of her personality to myself and other people. She's just quirky, I'd reason. She's in really good shape (the woman had abs when I was in college). She didn't get mad when I got busted for drinking in high school. I'd make her pose for photos and post them on Instagram like we were BFFs. She's not uninterested in being my mom, she's just delightfully weird!

As a devout follower of the church of manifestation, I'm familiar with the practice of delusional thinking. But convincing yourself that your mom will reconfigure their role in your relationship is very different than believing you'll get your dream job or apartment.

I've dumped this upon you in part to commiserate. I hope your misery enjoys my company. But my other goal is to demonstrate that, sometimes, moms don't change. Recognizing that might be a big part of getting yourself from acknowledgment all the way to acceptance.

WHY SOME MOMS STAY THE SAME

I wish this was the part where I start sounding like a TikTok creator at 1.5× speed explaining the one weird trick to get your mom to be different or better or different in a better way.

Sadly, there is a strong chance your mom will be like this forever—or at least until she wants to change. In some languages that roughly translates to "maybe, probably never."

Sorry if that came off as dismissive. This is really hard to say out loud, and I get how devastating it is to hear.

Whatever experiences or circumstances impacted your mom's parenting in the past may keep influencing her behavior indefinitely. If she's still struggling to cope with something from her past, it doesn't really matter how long ago the event or situation occurred. Any maladaptive coping mechanisms she developed as a result are hard to shake. If she's relied on them to keep her feeling safe for a long time, those coping mechanisms can be even more difficult to change.

So if your mom's maladaptive coping mechanisms have historically interfered with your relationship (and still are), the odds of your mom changing her ways are not good. Again, this sucks, and I'm sorry.

Your mom might not know how to function without, say, trying to control you or avoiding confrontation. She might feel extremely unwell in the face of negative feedback, emotional vulnerability, or just your feelings.

Yes, of course, it's possible for caregivers to have an epiphany and decide to shake up their life for the better and evolve emotionally. We'll talk more about what that would take in a minute.

But until they do, we have to acknowledge that whatever toxic coping strategy they've acquired might be final sale. Here's why.

Old habits are hard to break.

The ability to understand and manage emotions is a nonnegotiable when making meaningful changes within a relationship, says Whitney Goodman, therapist and founder of the Calling Home community and podcast. If your mom can't tolerate stress or fear without relying on an easy solve, she likely won't learn to use healthy coping mechanisms. That's the vicious cycle of emotional immaturity at work.

Again, people often develop maladaptive coping mechanisms after experiencing trauma early in life. But whether these tactics originated in childhood or later in life, the longer people depend on them to feel better, the more ingrained they become.

In childhood, those mechanisms might look like hiding under a bed, dissociating with TV, and taking fear or anger out on a sibling. When people don't find new, more emotionally mature ways to handle frightening stuff, stress, and anxiety, those habits can get "cemented" into our psyche and our behavior, Goodman explains.

On top of that, humans are wired to look out for threats. It's a safety feature that often backfires. For a caregiver with maladaptive coping mechanisms, any scenario that remotely looks or feels like the threatening ones from their childhood may trigger a reaction similar to the one they used as a kid. That's true whether the threat is actually there or not, says Goodman.

If Moms keep hitting that easy button, fending off scary things with the help of a messed-up coping strategy, it can create a feedback loop, affirming their fears and the need for that maladaptive coping tool to survive. They prove to themselves over and over again that they can't live without it. This mindset can make collateral damage, like their relationship with their kids, seem worth it.

Say your mom actively avoids talking about feelings, and you bring up something hurtful she did and how it made you feel. A mom who was never emotionally nurtured by her own parents might change the subject or shut you down to avoid that emotions-based convo. She doesn't know how to do feelings, so going there activates alarm bells.

Or, maybe your mom has always acted extremely entitled to your life (another sign of emotional immaturity). She wants you to have a certain career, produce an heir, partner up with a specific kind of person, look a certain way, and on and on.

If you rebel, she might verbally attack you, guilt-trip you, shame you, even yell. That's emotional manipulation, and it's a maladaptive coping mechanism too. Whatever it takes to get you back in line is fair game, according to her faulty coping system.

Addressing the problem is painful.

For lots of people, genuinely admitting fault and/or recalculating how they act when triggered can bring up painful emotions they've worked hard to avoid for maybe ever. Again, the goal of those behaviors is to avoid challenging feelings.

If caregivers really took the time to sit with their behavior and think about why they act that way, they might realize it stems from some pretty effed-up experiences (see: trauma). Or it might prove that their parents didn't have their back, care about their feelings, or treat them well, says Goodman. Sometimes maltreatment is cyclical.

For example, one of the common groups Goodman sees in her Calling Home community are Gen Zers, millennials, and young Gen Xers who are looking to emotionally connect with their parents but feel rejected. Those parents might act uninterested in their adult kids or avoid emotional intimacy with them.

That intolerance to closeness can happen when parents are emotionally immature, were emotionally neglected by their own parents, or are just unfamiliar with the whole feeling-your-feelings thing. In any of those cases, bonding might feel unsafe. So can investigating the reasons why it feels unsafe.

So, your mom may decide (consciously or not) that avoiding accountability forever is a solid option. Or, Goodman adds, she might mentally reframe her actions as positive. Like, *Yeah, I rarely told you I loved you, but look how independent you became!* It's not right, but you can see how the logic tracks.

They're too ashamed.

Another reason your mom might avoid engaging with awareness is a little thing called shame. Oh, and another one called guilt. If you've ever dabbled in those emotions, you know how hard it is to make peace with serious errors and move forward without the mistake montage replaying in your head. For a person who's rolled through life in a problematic way, that montage is years long, decades even.

If that's your mom, attempting to address her mess head-on can bring up shameful feelings and trigger her accountability shield. She might say, "How dare you come to me with this? Look at all the things I did for you," says Goodman. Shame and guilt, consider yourself successfully deflected.

Of course, there's also the possibility that her emotional immaturity prevents her from seeing a problem at all. She might even think her shitty behavior was warranted. *Screaming was the only way to get you to be quiet. Being hit is a rite of passage that makes you tough. Venting about relationship problems to a six-year-old was a bonding moment.* When they can't understand how their actions hurt you, even when you explain how, the problem doesn't exist—at least, in their mind.

WHY THEIR RELATIONSHIP WITH YOU ISN'T (ALWAYS) ENOUGH TO MOTIVATE THEM TO CHANGE

Here's a thing that sucks: Sometimes moms sacrifice their relationships with their kids to stay the course. They're not ready to address their past. They're not willing to live differently. They don't know how to change, and they're not open to trying. They just can't evolve.

Maybe you didn't need me to tell you that. Alas, the problem is bigger than both of us.

It's not that our moms don't love and care about us. They likely want us to be happy. Still, for some moms, those well wishes are just not enough to make moves, says Goodman. "As a therapist, I have to believe that everybody wants to change for the sake of their kid," she says. "But some people, for whatever reason, aren't going to—and I have to believe pain is at the center of that."

Pause for deep sighs.

While that truth certainly warrants a little compassion, Goodman offers another that exists alongside it: Some moms are unwilling to change because the existing dynamic works well for them. Engaging in a psychological glow-up for the sake of their relationship with their kid might require them to take some Ls.

Also, maybe your mom's not totally conscious that this relationship isn't as great for you as it is for her. If you said, "Hey, I don't think we have a healthy relationship," maybe she'd say, "You always take my phone calls, though! We see each other every Sunday! We connect over my feelings about your weight!" For her, those could be top-notch mother–adult child interactions. For you, they're why you dread seeing her name light up your phone.

Other moms might tell themselves there's no point in changing because they'd never be good enough. No matter what she did, she might think, you'd still hate her. Goodman says she's heard a lot of parents use language like this when talking about conflicts with their adult children. Those parents, she says, can be challenging to work with.

Some of these caregivers cling to the idea that they're the true victims. How that mentality benefits them depends on the person, but it could be another way to ditch accountability. If they had the power to change and improve their relationship, they might have to sit with the guilt and shame of their actions. If they could do better, they'd have to feel bad for not doing better in the past. That's tough.

WHAT IT WOULD TAKE FOR THEM TO CHANGE

To clarify, I'm not out here trying to villainize moms. It's just unhelpful to pretend trauma and pain don't also manifest in self-serving ways. Sometimes they do.

Whatever your mom went through though, she has free will just like the rest of us. Even if it feels laughable, we can choose to get it together and change the way we go through life. For the most part, we have the potential to take in feedback from people we value, swish it around our brains, and choose to drink it in. The same goes for our moms.

Sadly, not every mom is capable of reaching peak emotional maturity. As you know, starting points may vary, but Goodman says any mom can take steps to do better.

In general, "doing better" requires that your mom:

* **Be aware of the problem.** Telling her that there is a situation here could get her started, but she has to really *see* the problems in order to change.
* **Believe that doing something about the problem you've presented would improve her life in some way.** When she sees that changing her behavior is worthy of her time and energy, she could be more motivated to change.
* **Be resilient and willing to do the work.** To keep going when conflict arises or she's feeling extra uncomfortable, she has to persevere through challenging experiences.

Cool. But also, how? Logistically speaking, this process is slightly more involved. I'll give you the gist.

Moms need to be OK not being OK.

One of the biggest differences between moms who change and moms who don't is the capacity to withstand emotional pain, says Goodman. Moms have to endure hard feelings in order to admit they messed up, understand they made mistakes, and feel motivated to make up for it.

Moms have to combat toxic habits as they happen.

Embracing one's fuck-ups and making an effort to change takes guts. Your mom must be willing to spend as much time fixing said fuck-ups as she did making them. That's when the good stuff happens.

This is not an exaggeration, people. Goodman says moms need to literally spend as much energy fighting those maladaptive coping mechanisms as they did using them.

Moms (probably) have to start therapy.

Surprise! One of the best ways to endure the emotional meat grinder of owning up to mistakes and undo decades of trained responses is via therapeutic support, whether it's solo or in a group setting.

Therapy can help your mom get to the root of her reactions, bad behavior, and emotional immaturity. There, she'll reframe how she sees conflicts and triggers, and gain new tools for doing that. (That's like .0001 percent of the perks of therapy, but you get it.)

Support groups are kind of a secret hack for moms seeking a more emotionally mature lifestyle. That's because shame and guilt are major obstacles to changing one's ways—especially in a society that makes being a "bad mother" the ultimate insult. So if your mom can find other moms who mom like her (and want to change), she'll feel less alone. I don't know if you've heard, but a like-minded community can be the antidote to feeling embarrassed, lonely, and unworthy.

Goodman, who runs virtual groups as part of her Calling Home community, says, "Once somebody meets other people doing what they're doing, they say, 'Oh my gosh, I'm not the only one breaking this cycle. Something isn't wrong with me. There was something wrong with the system. And now that I see other people doing this, I can see that change is possible.'" That's a beautiful thing.

And then, of course, your mom will have to commit to doing her therapy homework, checking herself, and learning more about how her behavior impacts others.

When she gets to the point that she's noticing bad behavior and correcting it on her own, she's on her way to breaking harmful family cycles we know all too well, says Goodman.

Moms need a strong desire to change.

If you're feeling something right now, it might be hope. So let's go ahead and say the quiet part of all those criteria out loud: For this to work, your mom has to initiate changes on her own. Her emotional maturity, her choice.

It's normal, fine, and helpful to flag your grievances to your mom. If you haven't, maybe you should! But while you can share how her behavior made you feel and how she can remedy the situation, you *can't* force her to act.

If she really doesn't want to go to therapy, for instance, taking her will be futile. Giving her an ultimatum won't work either. In Goodman's experience, moms who enter therapy against their will won't change.

The moms who make meaningful shifts come in on their own. They join support groups for estranged adult children and take notes. They initiate those steps by themselves. "None of us fix every family curse, but I've seen people get really, really far," says Goodman.

Unfortunately, from what I can tell based on many, many conversations with mental health professionals, a "new year, new mom" scenario is not the norm. It takes energy and time for caregivers to recalculate the way they've been living for decades, admit fault, and make changes that stick. Not everyone is willing or able to risk it for the biscuit.

As much as it hurts, acknowledging that your mom may not change is how you can start moving toward acceptance.

CHAPTER 7

. . . And How to Accept That

Even with piles of anecdotal evidence and your own lived experience, you might feel better telling yourself that your mom is the exception to the rule. According to Big Mom, Inc., mothers are supposed to adore us more than anyone else ever. They are the epitome of love, care, and admiration. It's therefore normal to hold on to the fantasy that your relationship could become everything society promised—or at least closer to it.

It's also terrifying when our caregivers don't provide kindness, sensitivity, or empathy, notes Whitney Goodman, creator of Calling Home. When that happens, your brain is likely trying to do some serious emotional math. *If moms are supposed to treat their kids like they're the best thing to ever happen, and my mom doesn't, what the fuck does that say about me?*

That question is often at the root of our struggle to acknowledge mom's behavior for what it is, says Goodman.

And without first *acknowledging* the problem, the things we've spent the last chapter and all of part one talking about, we can't get any closer to acceptance (a.k.a. the whole point of all of this). That can seriously disrupt our lives.

When people hold out hope for their mom to become someone else, all that dissatisfied energy can be turned inward. You might base important decisions on what your mom thinks, says Goodman. You pursue a gig in accounting because your mom is an accountant. You don't date people below a certain income bracket because your mom will judge you. You don't move to a new city because your mom will be sad.

But these choices also might be smaller, like my mom-focused hypervigilance. Sure, the stakes of spending time on her hair and makeup or curating Ashley's Gift Guide (2010 Edition) aren't super high. Still, they're examples of the micro-control tactics I deployed in the hopes that Foxy would just learn. I do wonder where my time and energy could have gone if I hadn't spent it white-knuckling our relationship for decades. Alas, I thought that, with enough training, my mom would start to make me feel good.

At this point, though, I hope you can acknowledge that the problem is your mom, not you.

WHAT HAPPENS WHEN YOU STOP FIGHTING REALITY

Whether or not your mom has the desire and capability to change their behavior, accepting her as she is right now is the healthiest move you can make. It's the be-all, end-all of this healing thing.

Clinging to who you want her to be is understandable, but it just makes interactions with her, and life in general, much harder. Regardless of your mom's progress or lack thereof, taking care of *you* is all you can do.

It's true that my mom works out a lot, can talk at anyone who shows remote interest, and looks great with a blowout. It's also become obvious to me that those fun traits don't make our relationship any better.

There's nothing I want more for you and me than for this makeover montage to be a reality. As fun (?) as it is to sit here and write about moms and feelings and therapy, I would much rather be having deep conversations about life with the woman who gave birth to me.

Maybe she'd ask me for updates on my best friend's kids or tell me how a funny commercial reminded her of my sense of humor. That's not who she is, though, and that's not the relationship she set up for us. Becoming OK with that fact has literally changed everything for me. That's the beauty of acceptance, my babies.

HOW ACCEPTANCE HITS DIFFERENT

It's taken years of my life, thousands in therapy, and, apparently, a book deal, to get very comfortable with the reality of my relationship with my mom. Once I did, I started to move forward.

Yeah, I said years. Goodman says busting that Better Mom Fantasy is usually the hardest part of consolidating mom-based baggage—and it takes a while. For me, it was about six years, from starting therapy to setting very serious boundaries.

Before you chuck this book across the room and give up, hear me out: It gets better once you get started. The getting-started part often takes the most time.

When I finally believed my mom would continue to be the person she's been, there was nothing left to work for. It didn't always feel good to acknowledge that her version of a good relationship wasn't the same as mine, but it started to unravel the lies I'd told myself. With less of that fictional narrative playing on repeat, I could hear the facts.

This perspective shift is called "radical acceptance," and it's the most important part of moving on from your mom or moving forward *with* them in a healthy way, says Goodman.

In case you're not as deep in the psychological trenches as I am, radical acceptance is a skill used in dialectical behavioral therapy (a.k.a. DBT, if you're nasty). This idea, which has roots in Zen Buddhism, encourages people to accept reality as it is, including the things they don't like, along with their feelings around all that.

By the way, it's also perfectly fine to never say never. Your mom might have an epiphany and do a 180. Who knows! However, making peace with how she acts, the way she treats you, and your relationship with her *right now* is basically how you do radical acceptance.

If you don't accept who your mom is, you can't change your response to her. You still show up to Thanksgiving hoping this year she'll stop judging you. You wake up on your birthday wondering if she'll make the annual birthday call about herself again. You'll hear her scoff in your head more days than not.

When you see that she's doing her, and will continue to until further notice, you can change course. Do you want to keep ignoring your mom's eyerolls at dinner or do you want to call her out? Do you want to send Mom's call to voicemail on your birthday so you can enjoy a day without her shit getting you down? When you make different choices, you might notice that her power over you starts to fizzle out. The scoffs get quieter. They might even go away. That's why we worship in the house of acceptance.

"Your mom might be like this forever," says Goodman, "but you will not be like this forever." Your relationship with your mom and her behavior can change. Your life can too.

HOW TO GET SOME ACCEPTANCE

I mean, OK, that's the gist of radical acceptance, but there are actual steps for getting there. While the road can look a little different depending on who you ask, the following steps are based on dialectical behavioral therapy (DBT), created by psychologist and author Marsha M. Linehan, PhD.

DBT was developed to help people manage the symptoms of mental health conditions that cause big, disruptive feelings and sometimes lead to outbursts. Today, it's used to treat a variety of issues. It's also one of Goodman's favorite modalities for helping people deal with tricky family relationships.

DO YOU NEED AN ASSIST?

Speaking of therapy, now feels like a good time to recommend seeking out a mental health pro if you end up struggling with the process in this chapter. Helping people accept hard things is their whole deal. They can lend a hand with the tough feelings that come up through the process too.

Step 1: Notice whether you're fighting reality.

Think about how your mom behaves or treats you (both could be problematic, to be honest) 90 percent of the time. Is their rude sarcasm par for the course? Are their controlling tendencies always flipped on? Do most of your conversations revolve around them or their agenda? Do you feel judged or unsafe when you spend time together? (These are just a selection of mom-based issues. If your experience is different, it still counts!)

With that in mind, and being as realistic as possible, ask yourself:

* *Does part of me still think she'll be different?*
* *Am I still hoping she'll change?*
* *Do I think she should be different?*

Do not be alarmed if you answer yes to any or all of these questions. It's just more evidence that radical acceptance might be useful here.

As you're noodling on those prompts, notice the emotions associated with that my-mom-could-change fantasy. When you think about your relationship, do you feel bitter, pissed off, sad, ashamed, or other uncomfortable emotions? Maybe it's mixed. You might even have some fuzzy feels up in there, but if most of the emotions floating around feel bad—and you still believe your mom could change—you might be dabbling in toxic positivity.

Step 2: Say it with me: "It is what it is."

If you find yourself faking it, it's time to check yourself. Step 2 of practicing radical acceptance, per Dr. Linehan's *DBT Skills Training Handouts and Worksheets*, is to "remind yourself that the unpleasant reality is just as it is and cannot be changed."

If you're not reminded enough, take out your journal, a Google doc, or voice notes app and write a description of the "unpleasant reality" of this relationship. Whatever blank page you prefer is fair game (a trusted friend who gives blank page energy is good too).

Unlike Step 1, there's no need to ask yourself whether you're in denial about your relationship with your mom. The goal of this step is to see your mom for who they are, despite your best efforts.

Here, you're just venting out the facts. Be petty. It's fine. My own therapist encourages it.

That might look like "My mom rarely tries to make plans with me. The last time she did she also asked to borrow money. I tried to tell my mom how I appreciate when she reaches out, but she doesn't do it more often. Sometimes I wonder if she even heard me."

You're welcome to freestyle, but here are some prompts if you need them:

Reflect on the last time your mom behaved in a way that made you feel good.
How long ago was it?
When did it happen before then?

You're looking for a pattern here. How often *does* the good outweigh the bad? Is there any good at all?

Now think about all the things you've done to change that. Have you called out the behavior? If so, how did she respond? Was she defensive or receptive? How did that play out over time? Did anything change?

When she is nice to you, is it because you're putting up with her? Does it involve taking a hit, sucking it up, or putting your own needs aside for her comfort? Have you engaged in "pick me" behavior to get her attention, affirmation, or care? How often does that get the result you want? Are your actions sustainable?

Step 3: Consider why your mom is like this.

You could reread chapter two, or just spend some time thinking on the possible reasons your mom acts the way she does. You don't have to know her backstory or every trauma she experienced for this to work. Taking an educated guess is allowed. Blaming yourself is not.

In her books, Dr. Linehan makes it pretty clear that radical acceptance is not about excusing bad behavior or even being compassionate. But in my opinion, if you wanted to offer a little empathy to your mom here, you could. It might help you see that she's a person with flaws. It might also take more of the burden off your shoulders.

Step 4: Sit with that.

This is the part where we marinate in the acceptance juice. In her workbook, Dr. Linehan recommends finding ways to do this that involve your mind, body, and spirit. Maybe that means using a neutral affirmation when you find yourself wishing things were different.

Try one or more of the following:

* "My mom isn't someone I'd choose, and that's fine."
* "My relationship with my mom isn't healthy [close, loving, etc.], but I will be all right."
* "Spending time with my mom doesn't feel good, but I can take care of myself."

The point isn't to feel happy about your relationship with your mom or condone their actions. You're just getting comfortable with uncomfortable facts. That's the whole goal of acceptance.

There are some really helpful ways to practice acceptance or get closer to it. And I've got some activities lined up for that later. So don't get discouraged if these phrases aren't shifting you into acceptance mode. Again, coming to terms with what you've gone through and who your mom is can take years.

Step 5: Try something else.

One of the cool things about the radical acceptance process is that you don't have to complete one step before moving on to the next. If you can, that is very impressive. However, you don't want to spend months or years stuck on, say, the marination stage if you can make changes now.

And making changes is exactly what Step 5 is about. Dr. Linehan calls this practicing opposite action. First, think about how you'd interact with your mom if you believed that your dynamic would not change. List out all the things you would do differently. For example, let's say you normally stay quiet when your mom blames you for something you had no part in. Maybe, instead, you could drop a "Well, that was rude." Or ask her not to say stuff like that anymore. Then, do those things and see what happens.

You'll probably face pushback. And at first, breaking patterns might make you feel sad, guilty, or anxious. Still, when you continue to act in ways that align with the reality of your relationship, rather than the one you wish you had, you might start feeling more empowered. This was a hard one for me, and it might be for you as well.

When you're making choices based on what could be, it's hard to enjoy your life, says Goodman. "Acceptance sets you free to choose what's important to you," she adds. The short-term pain is worth the long-term gain.

If you're struggling to pinpoint what actions feel authentic to you, Goodman recommends asking yourself, *If this is who my mom is, what kind of relationship can I realistically have with her?*

You might decide to only answer her calls when you're in a good headspace, or to change the subject when she says something hurtful. You might limit how much time you spend together or the circumstances in which said hangs take place. The point is, you make the rules. Over time, when you're not constantly trying to please your mom, you'll begin to live your whole life differently. You could go after the job you really want, go back to school, date different people, or move somewhere new.

Step 6: Plan ahead.

Radical acceptance can help you feel less reactive to your mom's mess. When you go into an interaction with a clear view of your mom's patterns and the reality of your relationship, you can act defensively (in a good way). You can take a step back, think, *Yep, there it is*, and respond in a way that has "I saw this coming" energy.

The holidays are a lovely opportunity to employ this step. If you know that your mom will bring up politics at the dinner table and start crying when people disagree, how do you want to deal? Backing yourself into the bathroom and scrolling on your phone till things audibly cool down? Avoiding booze so you're less tempted to engage in a debate? Or just going on vacation instead of attending Thanksgiving dinner at all?

As they say, when you fail to plan (your reaction to your mom's unhinged behavior), you plan to fail (and freak the fuck out).

Step 7: Take care.

Learning to accept your mom, as she is, is really, really hard. I mean, you're confronting stuff you've avoided for a long time (a feat your mom likely hasn't even attempted). Go ahead and thank yourself for your service.

Also, be prepared to tend to yourself here. Dealing with The Mother can bring up all the feelings. When it does, your assignment is to feel those big emotions—not to fight them. The less you push them away, the easier they'll move along, and the quicker you'll rebound. More on that in the next chapter.

CHAPTER 8

How to Heal Through Grief

The highway to acceptance is full of potholes called grief. Maybe you remember it as the "running" part of my silly little track metaphor. It's the painful work we have to do to get from acknowledgment to that acceptance we talked about last chapter.

When you grieve, you come to terms with what's gone and find meaning in it. And if you trust the grief process, no matter how much it sucks, you'll find acceptance and a new normal. You'll reconfigure your assumptions about the world to include the loss and move forward within that reality. If that's not healing, I don't know what the hell is.

You can grieve a job you lost or an ex that dipped out—you know this. But the thing that helped me unlock a new level of growth was the realization that messed-up relationships with our moms are losses too.

You can grieve the hope of a stronger bond with the person who may have given birth to and/or raised you. You can grieve the idea of a person she'll never be. You can grieve what an unhealthy relationship with your mom took from you.

Thus, grieving may be the most important thing you can do to keep your mom's behavior from disrupting your life. Grief might even improve your relationship with her.

Here's my hypothesis: The point of grief is to accept the fact that you're missing something and to rework your outlook on life, knowing that thing will never be yours.

Accepting your mom, which we've talked about before (and will again), means accepting who she is, how she impacted you, and what being her kid means for your future. That's the whole goal here. Doing so enables you to finally shake off her grasp. Without her hold on your values, goals, and emotions, you're more likely to live the way you want. You're free to move about the cabin.

Again, to get to acceptance, we have to grieve what a dysfunctional relationship with our moms took from us. Without that step, we're just walking around feeling shitty and hoping things will somehow get better. Meanwhile, we contort ourselves to meet their expectations, minimize our emotions, and live in a version of reality that doesn't exist. None of that feels good.

From what I can tell, your relationship with your mom won't change if you don't. And grief—according to grief researchers—is all about change.

NON-DEATH LOSSES

As we've established, death isn't a prerequisite for loss (no disrespect to death). And there's actually a category for all those kinds of losses I just listed—plus others like them. Grief researchers call them non-death losses.

What's more, the good people who study grief have identified different kinds of non-death loss specific to how the loss occurred or how it feels—sometimes both.

We'll get into the details soon, but for now, know that you could experience all of these layers of loss at once.

Another thing: If you notice a ton of overlap among these terms, you're not wrong. What makes each kind of loss distinctive is the psychological theory it stems from. That's not super necessary for us to get into. I just wanted to give you a heads-up.

For our purposes, these vocab words are just more evidence that everything you're feeling, even if it's made no sense up to this point, is justified. It's OK to believe your complicated feelings about your mom.

Like I said, learning that you can lose a million little things that aren't people or jobs or money was a big deal for me. Just as calling out unhealthy caregiver behavior (i.e., abuse, parentifying, enmeshment) can deliver validation, so too can naming the types of loss you've experienced. Can you ever have enough of that? I say, *Nay.*

We could probably end the chapter with this fact: The losses you tallied up over the course of your relationship with your mom are real. However, drilling down to find your exact kind of loss adds more useful detail to your story. Getting extra specific enables you to look back on painful moments with your mom and acknowledge why they hurt so damn much. That newfound awareness can surface more events and emotions worth processing.

Ambiguous Loss

Ambiguous loss is an in-between kind of loss. It's the kind you might feel if someone you care about has dementia or ghosts you. The person isn't dead, but they're not in your life as they once were.

In the context of a dysfunctional relationship with your mom, this kind of loss could look like pining for closeness (even if you never had it) or wishing for a relationship where you have lots in common and you feel seen and appreciated. Your relationship with your mom isn't over, but it feels like something is missing. It doesn't make you feel the way you assume mom relationships should.

You could also feel the loss when your mom is physically present but emotionally unavailable. Say they pick you up from the airport, but don't seem excited to see you or ask what's new. Or maybe they help you move after a breakup but are MIA when you need a hug afterward. Maybe your mom's political outlook has seriously shifted in the last few years, and you miss the version of them you grew up with. That counts too.

When the thing you lost is fully present in your mind but physically unreachable, that's also a form of ambiguous loss. Maybe you blocked your mom's number after she pulled some crazy shit, but you still hear her retort to any given thought twenty times a day. Or perhaps it's Mother's Day, and you're not speaking to your mom right now (or vice versa).

Whatever the situation, Dr. Winokuer and Dr. Harris write in *Principles and Practice of Grief Counseling* that an ambiguous loss:

* Feels confusing
* Is misunderstood or not validated by other people
* Leaves you holding out hope things will change
* Triggers conflicting emotions like dread and relief or hope and hopelessness
* Makes you feel emotionally numb
* Feels isolating
* May never have closure

Nonfinite Loss

Nonfinite loss can likewise arise from an unhealthy relationship with your mom. Similar to ambiguous loss, nonfinite loss often doesn't have closure, is tough to describe, and can feel lonely. But this one typically sets in after something bad happens and goes on (like the name implies) indefinitely, writes Dr. Harris.

Perhaps you went through a really hard time and reached out to your mom for support only to be sent to voicemail. That could be a turning point where you realize they've never been a reliable source of emotional backup. Now, every time they ignore you, you can't unsee their emotional unavailability. The loss goes on for as long as you two stay in touch or even beyond.

Intangible Loss

When the thing that's gone missing or died is more of an abstract concept, like your identity, sense of control, well-being, or hope, that's an intangible loss, Dr. Harris explains.

Intangible losses are all valid, but they're also hard to convey to other people, hence the label. Nothing to see here, just mourning the loss of my ability to trust!

CALL IT WHAT YOU WANT—IT STILL SUCKS

Losing some aspect of your mom while they're alive and well can be disheartening, exhausting, depressing, and confusing. What do you have to be sad about if they call you every weekend? How can you feel bummed out when they're eager to help with your wedding? Why does spending a beach vacation with your mother make you feel nauseous?

The answer: Your mom spends most of those calls talking about herself. Your mom is using your wedding to flex her power over you. Your mom has a history of dropping judgey comments about your body.

In each of those examples, you're hit with a loss. In the first, you've lost the dream of a mom who's curious about your life and interested in you as a person (ambiguous loss). In the second, you've lost your sense of agency over an important life event (intangible loss). And in the third, you've lost your ability to trust that your mom is a safe space (nonfinite loss).

No matter what form it takes, a loss is a loss—and it hurts.

CHRONIC SORROW

To process any loss, we have to grieve. Depending on the circumstances, that grief can come in different forms.

When you get fired, the loss is finite. You had that job and now you don't. When you're grieving, say, the idea of a mom you never had or a childhood you deserved, the loss is ongoing. It never really goes away, but it hits hardest on their birthday, your birthday, Mother's Day, when something big happens to your family, when your high school friend's mom asks about your mom in the freezer aisle of the grocery store. There's no escape.

This experience is called chronic sorrow, and it's a type of grief associated with all those hard-to-pin-down losses in dysfunctional parent–child relationships. This form of grief happens any time there's a discrepancy between what's actually going on and what you're holding out hope for, according to psychotherapist Susan Roos, PhD, author of *Chronic Sorrow: A Living Loss*. At every turn, you're confronted by what is and how you wish things were.

In the thick of my chronic sorrow situation, I was on edge any time mom-related stuff came up. A running buddy, work friend, or rando at a party would say something endearing about their mom with a half-smile and an eyeroll—"Moms, right?"

Then I'd think, *Their relationship seems healthy and normal. Mine isn't. They have no idea that I'm secretly defective.* Still, I'd play it off like *Yes, I very much relate to this "we have moms who care about us so much we're embarrassed about it" narrative.* "Moms! Right!"

Whenever the societal trope of momkind's unwavering love crossed my path, I'd get lost. I'd go inward, comparing my experience to those examples. More often than not, I felt physically dirty and lesser than anyone with a good relationship with their mom. The word "dysfunctional," though applicable to my situation, made me feel icky. I wanted my life to be like Lizzie McGuire's, but it wasn't.

Solo interactions with Foxy triggered my chronic sorrow too. When I moved into my dorm room freshman year, the resident advisors asked parents to secretly write letters to their kids, which the advisors would then deliver later. Cute idea.

I opened mine from my mom, hoping for something mushy that told me how she'd loved watching me grow up and how excited she was for me to start college. Instead, it said something along the lines of "Don't put yourself in a bad situation" (read: don't get yourself assaulted).

After moving to New York City, I told my mom that some of my equally broke friends got care packages from their parents. I asked if she could send me one (I learned long ago that care and attention require solicitation). A couple of weeks later, a box showed up with cans of food from her pantry that would have otherwise ended up in a hunger drive bin. There was also a half-eaten bag of tortilla chips.

Years later, amid wedding planning, my mom said she wanted to walk down the aisle with my dad and me. Her parents did the same at her ceremony. And Foxy was "the mother of the bride, after all." When I offered up my future husband Sean to escort her instead, she replied, "That's fine, as long as someone important is with me."

Over time, the chronic part of my sorrow got worse. I started to dread her calls. If I answered, I'd be bummed out for hours after I hung up. If I avoided them, I'd feel bad and face backlash from her via text or other family members repeating her side of the story back to me.

Thirty seconds after one otherwise uneventful phone call with Foxy, I burst into tears. Sean was very confused. So was I.

Looking back, this was some motherfucking grief. Though I didn't know it at the time, I met many of the criteria for chronic sorrow, per Dr. Harris and Dr. Winokuer in *Principles and Practices of Grief Counseling*:

* I had "lost" some important parts of an attachment figure (Foxy).
* There was a big ol' gap between my expectation for normal life (a mom who had my back, cared about my feelings, and was interested in me) and my reality (half a bag of tortilla chips and a can of green beans).
* I held out hope that—with enough careful instruction—Foxy could figure out how to be my mom.
* Internal thoughts and external experiences triggered a sense of unavoidable sadness.
* That sadness had periods of highs and lows but never really went away.
* I was anxious about my interactions with Foxy and the lack thereof.
* My dysfunctional relationship with my mom never ended, so the grief lived on too.

For my people who've been feeling a lot of feelings about their moms for as long as they can remember, I hope this new vocab word helps. Categorizing many of the complex emotions related to my mom as part of chronic sorrow made them seem manageable. When I didn't have to justify what I felt, I had more space to process those emotions. Maybe it will do the same for you.

DISENFRANCHISED GRIEF

Even if *you* fully understand your feelings of loss and their origin story, our culture can't compute them. When someone dies, people send flowers, we have ceremonies and rituals, and, if you're lucky, you can take bereavement leave from work. With time and support, it gets easier to move forward without getting stuck in the big feelings of loss.

But there's no death certificate for a complicated relationship with your mom or condolence card for the loss of unconditional maternal support. Explaining an ambiguous loss and its impact on your life can leave the most well-meaning friends perplexed.

There's even a name for when a loss isn't fully recognized by your people or society in general: disenfranchised grief. And it can apply to dysfunctional relationships with our moms, too, says grief researcher Dr. Neimeyer, who we met in chapter five.

As the "disenfranchised" bit implies, the term describes grief that is hard for other people to understand or is stigmatized in some way. Some might say that the grieving process doesn't apply to your situation. You might struggle to justify your grief too.

Because we're all wired to crave acceptance and connection, how society and our social circles validate the mom loss (or don't) matters. If no one gets why you're so upset, you can't easily talk about the relationship with others. If there's no system in place to help you through your grief, there's no designated time and place for people to offer sympathy, writes Kenneth J. Doka, PhD, in *Non-Death Loss and Grief.* Without those pillars of mourning, it's hard to understand where emotions like sadness, loneliness, anxiety, or even depression are coming from. That leads to shame, insecurity, and confusion. Then, instead of seeking help to process your extremely valid mom-based loss, you deny that anything is wrong. You're just being dramatic. Other people have it so much worse. Never mind!

That's what can make grieving your relationship with your mom challenging and drawn out. Because your loss is ambiguous, nonfinite, and intangible, it's outside the norm of what people (aside from grief researchers) consider a loss. But that doesn't make it less painful.

In fact, a niche loss, such as the motherfucked kind, often hurts more and lasts longer. In *Non-Death Loss and Grief*, Dr. Harris explains that disenfranchised grief is compounded by the social pressure—explicit or not—to get the fuck over it (my paraphrase) and also by loneliness. When others don't believe or validate you after a loss, you're missing out on an important part of the grieving process.

Finding comfort in community helps us understand a loss. That's especially helpful when the loss involves a relationship society puts on a pedestal. If your social circles agree that it's very reasonable and appropriate for you to be upset, you can process feelings and move forward more easily. It's not a cure, but it makes feeling bad more bearable.

HOW DISENFRANCHISED IS YOUR GRIEF?

If you're looking for a little more proof that what you're actually experiencing is disenfranchised grief, this quiz (adapted from a questionnaire for the Social Meaning in Life Events Scale developed by Dr. Neimeyer and his colleagues*) could serve as an extra dose of validation. This isn't a diagnostic tool or anything, but it is a source of objective affirmation from

* Developed by Benjamin W. Bellet, Jason M. Holland, and Robert A. Neimeyer, and published in 2018 in *Death Studies*.

researchers who study disenfranchised grief. It can help you get a sense of how much social validation and support you're receiving (or not) for this loss.

Instructions

For each statement in the two sections below, circle the number that aligns with your perspective right now. When you're done, add up the numbers in each section and divide them by the number of questions in that section. You can come back to this to track how your perspective changes over time.

Part 1: Social Invalidation

1. **I worry that if I share too much about my relationship with my mom, people might see me differently.**

   strongly disagree 1 2 3 4 5 strongly agree

2. **I have difficulty getting people to understand how hard this has been for me.**

   strongly disagree 1 2 3 4 5 strongly agree

3. **I would like to talk about my relationship with my mom, but I don't think others would understand.**

   strongly disagree 1 2 3 4 5 strongly agree

4. **My relationship with my mom is too complicated to talk about.**

   strongly disagree 1 2 3 4 5 strongly agree

5. **I avoid sharing the story of this relationship with others to avoid their criticism and judgment.**

   strongly disagree 1 2 3 4 5 strongly agree

6. **I keep the details of my relationship with my mom to myself because they don't quite make sense.**

   strongly disagree 1 2 3 4 5 strongly agree

7. **I feel more distant from others when I talk to them about this relationship.**

   strongly disagree 1 2 3 4 5 strongly agree

8. **No one really understands what my relationship with my mom means to me.**

   strongly disagree 1 2 3 4 5 strongly agree

9. **I feel like my role in this relationship is often misunderstood by other people.**

   strongly disagree 1 2 3 4 5 strongly agree

10. **I feel more confused about this relationship after I talk to other people about it.**

    strongly disagree 1 2 3 4 5 strongly agree

11. **I feel more uncomfortable around people because of my relationship with my mom.**

    strongly disagree 1 2 3 4 5 strongly agree

12. **This relationship only makes sense to others if I leave some of the details out.**

    strongly disagree 1 2 3 4 5 strongly agree

13. **I don't want to burden others by talking about my relationship with my mom.**

    strongly disagree 1 2 3 4 5 strongly agree

14. **Because of my relationship with my mom, I don't feel like I fit in with other people.**

    strongly disagree 1 2 3 4 5 strongly agree

15. **There are few people I can confide in about this relationship.**

    strongly disagree 1 2 3 4 5 strongly agree

TOTAL SCORE ____ DIVIDED BY 15 = ____

Part 2: Social Validation

16. **Talking to other people about my relationship with my mom has brought some clarity to the situation.**

    strongly disagree 5 4 3 2 1 strongly agree

17. **Opening up about my relationship with my mom has helped bring resolution to the situation.**

    strongly disagree 5 4 3 2 1 strongly agree

18. **Talking about my relationship with my mom has helped me make sense of it.**

    strongly disagree 5 4 3 2 1 strongly agree

19. **When I tell people about my relationship with my mom, I believe they feel closer to me.**

    strongly disagree 5 4 3 2 1 strongly agree

20. **Other people have shared with me useful perspectives on this relationship.**

    strongly disagree 5 4 3 2 1 strongly agree

21. Sharing my story about this relationship has brought about greater compassion in others.

strongly disagree 5 4 3 2 1 strongly agree

22. Others can learn something valuable by hearing me talk about my relationship with my mom.

strongly disagree 5 4 3 2 1 strongly agree

23. I have comfortably shared my own private story about this relationship with others.

strongly disagree 5 4 3 2 1 strongly agree

24. The way I've handled my relationship with my mom has served as a positive example for others in my life.

strongly disagree 5 4 3 2 1 strongly agree

TOTAL SCORE ____ DIVIDED BY 9 = ____

Results

Section 1: Social Invalidation

Your social invalidation score is meant to get a sense of how much your grief is being dismissed, judged, or minimized by people in your social circles (aka how disenfranchised your grief is).

> **If your social invalidation score (your total for questions 1 through 15 divided by 15) is between 4 and 5:** Invalidation is likely. As a result, you might be feeling awkward, messy, or dramatic about the situation with your mom and the emotions it brings up. But that doesn't mean you *are* those things. You're just in need of social support (more on how to get it under "Now What?").

If your social invalidation score (your total for questions 1 through 15 divided by 15) is between 1 and 3: Don't let this sexy score invalidate your disenfranchised grief experience. A dysfunctional relationship with your mom is a loss that society doesn't always understand (if it did, we wouldn't be here doing this). And that's the definition of disenfranchised grief. Your low score doesn't mean your grief isn't disenfranchised. It means you're feeling more comfortable with that grief, and that can help you grow from this loss. You can't hear me, but I'm clapping for you.

Section 2: Social Validation

Your social validation score is meant to reflect how much your social support system acknowledges, accepts, and supports you through this loss.

If your social validation score (your total for questions 16 through 24 divided by 9) is between 1 and 3: It seems you've found people who get what you're going through. Head down to the "Now What?" section to see how you can make the most of these strengths!

If your social validation score (your total for questions 16 through 24 divided by 9) is between 4 and 5: It seems like you're having a hard time connecting with people who understand what you're going through or just offer their support. That's tough. But maybe reading these prompts can serve as goals to work toward as you process your grief. Read more on how to do that in the next section!

Now What?

If you've been DIY-ing your grief process, here's how to use all that emotional data you just collected to find more support:

Find what's working (and do more of it). Look back at statements 1 through 16 from Part 1. Are there any where you circled a 1 or a 2? If so, those are probably the moments or situations you feel most confident expressing your feelings about your mom. Let's max those out, shall we?

For example, say you strongly disagree that there are few people you can confide in about this relationship (question 15). In other words, there are several people you can comfortably vent about your mom with. Make a note of who those people are. Is it a friend whose mom causes similar kinds of ruckus? Is it your partner who sees this stuff play out in real time? Whoever they are, ask if they're down for regular mom-vent sessions as you process your grief.

If that feels like too much, consider joining something like a virtual support group for children of emotionally immature parents. (Yes—those exist!) There, you can share your story with people who get it. If you haven't already, find a therapist who can help you deepen your understanding of the situation. They could add 'roids to this existing strength.

Then, take a look at Part 2 and notice anywhere you circled a 4 or 5. Can you make the most of these situations, since they already seem to be working? Maybe test the waters to see if you can comfortably chat about your relationship with your mom with more people (#23). Find someone you trust, tell them a little, and see how you feel after.

Consider what's holding you back. Take another look at Part 1 and find any statements where you circled a 4 or 5. Then, look at Part 2, noticing where you circled a 1 or 2. Those indicate where your struggles may be keeping you from making sense of your relationship with your mom. (You definitely knew this.) That means they're also an ~opportunity for growth~ (in corporate annual-review speak).

For each of those statements, ask yourself (where it makes sense): *How could this be easier? Is this really true? Why do I believe this?* For example, if you agree that you "avoid sharing the story of this relationship with others to avoid their criticism and judgment" (question #5), think about who makes you feel judged. Has anyone criticized you for sharing your struggles with your mom in the past? Is it possible that other people might not react the same way? Or maybe this fear isn't backed up by any real experience. If that's the case, could you dip your toe into having that convo with someone trustworthy, open minded, and kind?

You can also dig into your answers via journaling or working with a therapist. You could even bring your answers to this questionnaire right to your mental health professional of choice.

Address what you're unsure about. For questions where you circled a 3, you're basically saying that you could go either way: Sometimes you feel like people won't get it, and sometimes you don't. It could depend on the person, the day, or the social context.

The cool part is you can address these statements as opportunities. Say you landed on a 3 for "When I tell people about my relationship with my mom, I believe they feel closer to me" (#19). Think about a time when you most agreed with this statement. Did you meet someone new who shared their latest mom saga? Did sharing your story help you bond a little more? If so, how can you lean into that strength and find closeness with other people who understand what you're dealing with? Maybe it's joining a support group or casually dropping "I'm not that close with my mom" into conversation (I mean, within reason). People who relate might say, "Yep, same," opening the door to new relationships where you can share this part of yourself.

Then, consider a time when you really disagreed with that statement. When did telling someone about your mom add distance? Who was it? Is it possible that they're just not a safe space? Could someone else react differently if you got vulnerable about your mom? Maybe!

HOW TO GRIEVE

All right, so now you know more about what an unhealthy relationship with your mom can take from you, and how those specific, often unrecognized losses can be challenging to move through without social support, understanding, and validation. Processing disenfranchised grief and chronic sorrow requires us to have our own backs. Of course, that doesn't always come naturally—especially if you often second-guess whether your feelings are warranted.

If you're struggling to trust that your feelings make sense, take it from someone who recently acquired several psychological textbooks on the topic: Your grief is real. For my friends who exist on the less extreme end of the mom-relationship spectrum, hi! You get to grieve too.

Say you have a very nurturing mom you love to spend time with, but they often project their body insecurities onto you. Whether they're envious or judgmental, the loss here could be your self-esteem. You've also kissed the ability to *not* think about your body goodbye. All of that is worth working through.

Whatever the case, allow me to franchise your grief by welcoming all losses into this space. Following are the steps you can take now (or whenever) to start sorting through your grief. How you go about doing that is totally up to you. While these steps imply a sequence, feeling your feelings doesn't always happen in a linear way. You might move back and forth between a few of the steps before hencing forth.

Also, since chronic sorrow is . . . chronic, you could finish Step 6, only to be confronted by a different angle of your grief you hadn't encountered yet. Then, it's back to the beginning. Cue the track analogy from chapter five. (If the infinity loop of grief feels overwhelming, I understand. I hope knowing there are steps for managing it brings some solace.)

Here we go!

Step 0.5: Name your grief.

We've been talking about this since chapter three, but it's worth repeating: You're probably not being dramatic or blowing things out of proportion. Grieving a dysfunctional relationship with your mom is a real thing, and you're likely dealing with it right now.

This reminder is brought to you by psychology: Mental health clinicians have reported that putting a name to the experience of grief, like chronic sorrow and disenfranchised grief, can lead to "immediate relief and comfort," writes Dr. Roos in *Non-Death Loss and Grief.*

So write this down, say it out loud to no one, or tell it to someone who gets you: "I just found out I'm probably dealing with chronic sorrow and disenfranchised grief. Have you heard about this shit before?" You can also just reread the first half of this chapter and think about how those vocab words apply to you.

Step 1: Name your losses and how they show up.

Calling out the consequences of your dysfunctional relationship with your mom is just as powerful as putting a name to the kind of grief you are experiencing. By focusing on what's missing or what never existed in the first place, you're putting words to an experience that's often unspoken, write Dr. Neimeyer and Lara Krawchuk, LCSW, in *Non-Death*

Loss and Grief. It's another way to reassure yourself that the sadness and mental spirals are understandable reactions.

You can start by naming what I like to call The Big Loss, also known as your primary loss. Try asking yourself: *What am I missing out on?* The first thing that comes to mind is probably your primary loss. That could be a healthy relationship with your mom, or having the kind of mom you always hoped for, or having any relationship with your mom at all. It could be all of that.

You also need to acknowledge the losses stemming from the primary loss, explains Dr. Neimeyer. These are called secondary losses, and they're all the ways that big missing piece manifests in your life now. It's the "chronic" part of chronic sorrow and the "nonfinite" in nonfinite loss.

Feel free to make a list and see them all written out. Your secondary losses could include worrying about having kids (or messing up the ones you've got). It could be having an awful time during your frat's annual mom's weekend, or being unable to trust those closest to you. One of mine was losing the last night of my bachelorette weekend to sobbing on a couch, venting about Foxy.

That secondary loss list could be long, but you don't have to account for every single one. It'll still be useful in gaining more awareness of how this relationship impacted your life and accounting for the ways you've been grieving so far.

Whether you made an actual list or not, see if you pick up on any themes among your losses. Getting a sense of those recurring issues can help you understand how to address it, says Dr. Neimeyer. (We'll circle back to that problem-solving stuff.) Maybe feeling unseen is a real hardship for you in your relationship with your mom and beyond. For me, feeling like I'm totally on my own without support still pops up, especially in stressful situations. But don't worry if you can't suss out a consistent narrative here. Maybe it will come to you in the next step, or maybe it won't! Either way, voicing the things that hurt you is a win.

For those struggling to believe secondary losses are in fact losses, try labeling them with one of the types of loss we talked about earlier. Again, one loss can fit into multiple categories:

* Ambiguous loss (a loss that remains unclear and without resolution)
* Nonfinite loss (enduring losses that are often caused by a negative life event; the loss has an ongoing physical or mental presence)
* Intangible loss (a loss that's often hidden, abstract, or existential—for example, loss of trust, identity, or a sense of control)

Step 2: ID your emotions.

Maybe you've heard the pro-feelings propaganda: Feel it to heal it! Name it to tame it! Sounds cute and catchy, but it's painful and sucks.

It's hard to feel all the emotions related to our moms. We get a lump in our throats when we think about our history with them. We feel a pit in our stomachs when we see their missed call. We notice the weight of guilt when we don't want to call them back.

You may feel like the poor guy from the boardgame *Operation*, getting zapped with big feelings at random. But spending time with those jolts—rather than pretending everything is fine—can be worth it. There are lots of reasons why paying attention to your emotions is helpful when your relationship with your mom is messy. The first, and maybe most significant, is the consequence of *not* doing it.

When we ignore our feelings or find some way to subdue them, they often come back up. That sounds a bit amateur life coach-y, but I come bearing psychology. In his book *Permission to Feel: The Power of Emotional Intelligence to Achieve Well-Being and Success*, emotion researcher Marc Brackett, PhD, writes that our feelings influence us most when we let them fly under the radar, undetected.

When we smush those emotions deep down or ignore them completely, they can evolve into a new, stronger, attention-grabbing form. Then, even if we don't realize it, those feels impact how we exist, writes Dr. Brackett, who's also the founding director of the Yale Center for Emotional Intelligence and a professor in the Child Study Center at the Yale School of Medicine. "The really powerful emotions build up inside us, like a dark force, that inevitably poisons everything we do, whether we like it or not," he writes.

Ignoring our feelings also means we're ignoring pieces of ourselves, explains Dr. Neimeyer. If those emotions are rooted in feeling unseen or dismissed by your mom, the invisibility compounds. It's like telling yourself, *No, your feelings are wrong. Why are you making this a thing?*

Our emotions signal to us that there's a problem. That's their job. And when you get all up in those feelings—sitting with how they show up, naming them, getting comfortable being uncomfortable—you can start working to solve the issue.

Emotions aren't annoying distractions. In the context of a dysfunctional relationship with your mom, they're a cheat code for achieving acceptance—the thing we've set out to do here.

When you're grieving a relationship with your mom, emotions tell you what you don't have, what you wish you did, and what you want to do about it, Dr. Neimeyer explains. To get started, you just have to "name them and claim them" (the mental health world has quality taglines).

The emotion that comes up most often in a conflictual relationship, such as the one with your mom, is anger, says Dr. Neimeyer. It asserts boundaries and keeps people at a distance.

While recognizing that feeling is gold-star, emotionally mature behavior, being pissed off is just the candy shell covering grief's gooey center.

Grief, in emotion form, often shows up as a mix of sadness and longing for something we lost or never had. But that's not the only shape it takes. When you're experiencing grief, you might also feel anxiety and a loss of identity, says Dr. Neimeyer. Furthermore, some grief research suggests that experiencing an ongoing ambiguous loss can also make us feel distracted, withdrawn, needy, irritated, or even numb.

With ambiguous loss, the kind that has you fantasizing about what could be while grieving what is, you might often feel hopeful that things can change—and disappointed when the same stuff keeps happening. Conflicting emotions are par for this course.

"Grief has many different dimensions," says Dr. Neimeyer. By noticing your grief-related emotions, you'll find it easier to address the reasons they're coming up in the first place, he adds.

THE *MOTHERF*CKED* FEELINGS BINGO CARD

Because there are so many emotions specific to mom grief, especially the disenfranchised, chronic kind, I bring you an interactive moment.

This BINGO card contains really specific feelings that can come up during this kind of grief process, based on my interviews with experts and my own experiences.

Use your phone to take a photo of the card and keep it tucked away in your photos app. Then, when those big emotions come up, check your card to see if it's a match (or pop it in the free space). If it is, cross it off.

If turning this into a game feels like too much of an ask, that's cool. The point is to spot your feelings when they come up (unexpectedly or not), so you can attend to them. You can do that anytime.

B	I	N	G	O
Needy	Wishful longing	Hopeful delusion	Annoyed by everything	General numbness
Righteous anger	Something big and nameless	Really, deeply sad	Heavy-hearted	So lost
Completely exhausted	Nobody-gets-me lonely	Insert your own emotion here	On edge	Unexplainable guilt
Sad + nostalgic	Insecure	Make-it-make-sense frustration	Actually depressed	Primal rage
Distracted by my thoughts	Mostly confused	Pure disap-pointment	Tainted or broken	Uninterested in anything

Step 3: Get into your grief.

Knowing that chronic sorrow never goes away, that we just get better at managing it, probably would have brought grief's life-changing powers into my life much, much sooner.

I had a lot of therapy sessions where my mental health wizard encouraged me to prioritize being sad. So, once every six months, I'd spend an hour in the bathtub listening to (probably) Taylor Swift and soaking in my despair. I called it progress. But grieving isn't a thing you can time like an oil change. Sadly (literally), you may have to integrate it into your day-to-day life to feel the effects.

More about me: The day after a long-procrastinated convo with my mom in which I told her about herself, I was shocked how *not* healed I felt. During the call, she struggled to see her part in our distant relationship or agree to make changes. Afterward, I cried all the way to hot yoga and all the way back—a respectable thirty minutes of sadness, I thought. I went to bed feeling accomplished. I finally expressed the problems I saw, stood up for myself, attempted to set boundaries, and grieved. Success, no?

Nope. Not success. I woke up feeling what I assume was depression. A heavy, dark, unamused cloud followed me for weeks. I couldn't figure out why. I'd named the problematic behavior! I'd multitasked commuting and being sad about what our relationship will never become! *Dusts off hands.* Where was my acceptance and motherfucking healing?

It turns out that, in order to grow, I had to feel my grief-based feelings regularly. Without that consistency, I couldn't get past my intrusive mom thoughts, accept the relationship as it was, or figure out what I wanted to do about it. And, praise be to grief researchers, there is a very specific way to go about this.

The process is called the dual process model. The "dual" in "dual process" means we have two main objectives: to grieve the thing we lost and to go about our lives as normally as possible. Going back and forth between these states, the first of which is called loss orientation and the second of which is called restoration orientation, can help us feel the feelings, find acceptance, and make positive changes. The grief researchers who coined this model, Margaret Stroebe, PhD, and Henk Schut, PhD, refer to the process of alternating grieving and living as a "dosage of grieving," which I love.

Grief researchers hypothesize that oscillating between grief mode and life mode helps us revise how we see the world. It lets us incorporate the reality of what *is* into our idea of what the world *should be*. We fold the experience of loss into our lives so we can accept what's gone and make choices from that new perspective.

That's how we can start to accept the dysfunction in our relationships with our moms and decide what to do about it. It can also enable us to go about everyday life without heavier feelings intruding. To be clear, those emotions don't go away, but they become less invasive—and less likely to swamp you when you're just trying to watch *Mamma Mia!* in peace.

In life mode, you're going about your regularly scheduled programming. Sometimes that means distracting yourself from grief with work, school, laundry, and coffee runs. It could also look like sensing an oncoming grief attack and deciding to deal with those feelings later (and actually doing that).

Other times, life mode means rebuilding your reality, making room for the things you lost, or becoming aware of new possibilities while going about your day-to-day. Those nondistraction activities, where you're living and also addressing the loss somehow, help integrate losses into the way you see the world.

For example, you might be in the shower, washing your hair and thinking about what you've accomplished without the support of your mom. Or you might be out for a walk with your dog and realize you don't need a close relationship with your mom to have a really beautiful life. Two birds, one dog. In life mode, you're distracting yourself from what you lost (as we discussed earlier) *or* doing your thing while also coming to terms with what's missing.

In grief mode, you're (obviously) going deep into the grief. It's got your full attention. This immersive experience is when you're returning to the anger, depression, fatigue, anxiety, frustration, hopelessness, or whatever feelings your grief delivers, and rolling around in them.

Dr. Neimeyer says that regularly taking a little time to be with your losses and how they make you feel can lead to acceptance. Ideally, you've planned this time. Sometimes, though, loss catches you out of the blue, and before you know it, you're projectile grieving. It happens, says Dr. Neimeyer. Still, the more you practice the grief mode/life mode vibe shift, the more the grief attacks should diminish.

When scheduling your date with grief, find a time and place to be alone. It could be the shower, your bedroom with the door locked, on the couch, or lying on your kitchen floor. Whatever feels safe and sound works.

It's not always easy to activate those painful feelings on cue. (Hello, my fellow emotional avoidance experts.) If you can relate, try coaxing your grief out by offering it a little treat. That could be a playlist that hits you where it hurts (never underestimate the power of a breakup ballad in any circumstance) or a movie that does the same. You could also spend time with your camera roll or old family albums. Journaling out what feels bad about your relationship with your mom works too. Whatever brings on the emotions you've been avoiding is fair game.

When the emotions hit, let them. You don't have to spend all day in it. Just be OK with not being OK (as the old Pinterest quote goes) for as long as you can or want to. I should say that longer periods of grief mode won't necessarily result in faster progress. The dual process model is more about getting used to grieving *while* living than enduring the sads for as long as possible.

Then, it's time to process. By acknowledging your emotions, explains Dr. Neimeyer, you're in a better place to ask, *What would make me feel better?* Maybe that's journaling, starting an art project, wrapping yourself in a blanket, or screaming the lyrics to "All Too Well (10 Minute Version) (Taylor's Version)" as many times as you want. (I've included some other options later in this chapter, if you're interested in my wares.) However you self-soothe, it's called self-compassion, and it works.

Once your self-allotted grief time is up, it's back to life mode. Unfortunately, this transition can be rough. As we've established, I'm a person who avoided grief for a long time. When I first started entering grief mode, I couldn't just exit the pool after diving headfirst into my emotions. I had to linger in the shallow end a bit. I'd cancel plans, keep listening to sad songs, and wallow until it was time for bed. This is not sustainable. I do not recommend.

To ease the grief hangover, plan something to look forward to. And it doesn't have to be A Thing. Grab a fancy coffee with a friend or by yourself, go for a run, open that bag of Hot Cheetos while catching up on garbage TV. You get the idea.

To recap: The dual process model entails living your life and noticing the grief-y feelings when they come up. Attend to them right away when you can or make a plan to come back to them when you get a minute. (Just don't keep them waiting, because they *will* find you.) Then, when your grief work is complete, swing back into routines and obligations. Live, grieve, love.

When your mom becomes less present in your brain and you feel less affected by the old triggers, you'll know you're doing it right, says Dr. Neimeyer.

Just a heads-up: Spending quality time with your emotions might give you more information about what you've lost, so feel free to pop back into Steps 1 and 2 to add to your list whenever you have a grief epiphany.

CHOOSE YOUR OWN SAD-VENTURE

So you're ready to do some grief-mode shit but aren't sure about the best modality for your grieving needs? Welcome. I'm pleased to assist.

I've created a manual algorithm to guide you, based on factors like your location, your schedule, and the amount of time since your last grief attack.

Just answer the questions in the following chart to find the ideal grieving activity for your very important, very busy life (or skip this part and just pick whatever looks good). Bon appetit!

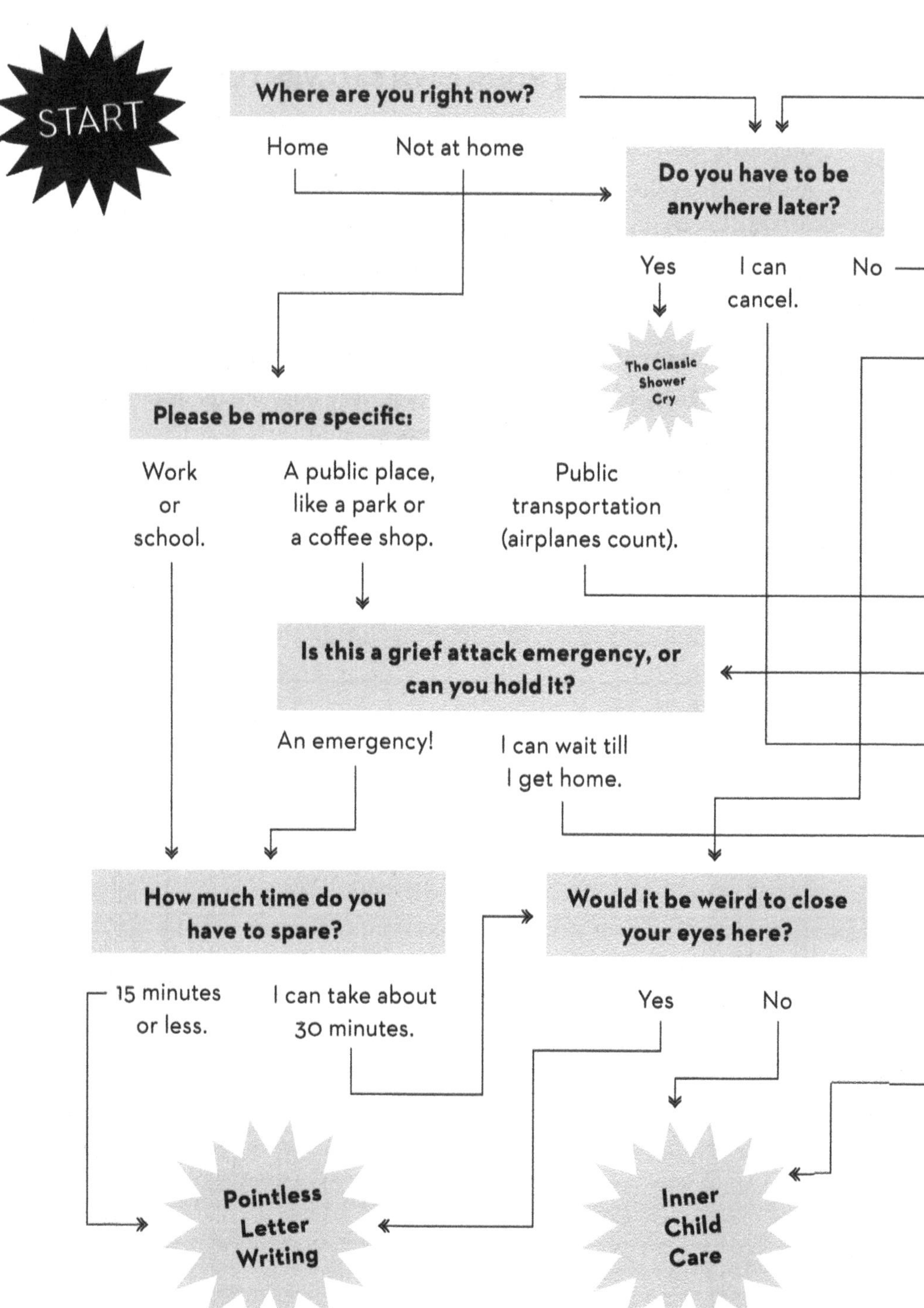

START
Where are you right now?
Home
Not at home
Do you have to be anywhere later?
Yes
I can cancel.
No
The Classic Shower Cry
Please be more specific:
Work or school.
A public place, like a park or a coffee shop.
Public transportation (airplanes count).
Is this a grief attack emergency, or can you hold it?
An emergency!
I can wait till I get home.
How much time do you have to spare?
15 minutes or less.
I can take about 30 minutes.
Would it be weird to close your eyes here?
Yes
No
Pointless Letter Writing
Inner Child Care

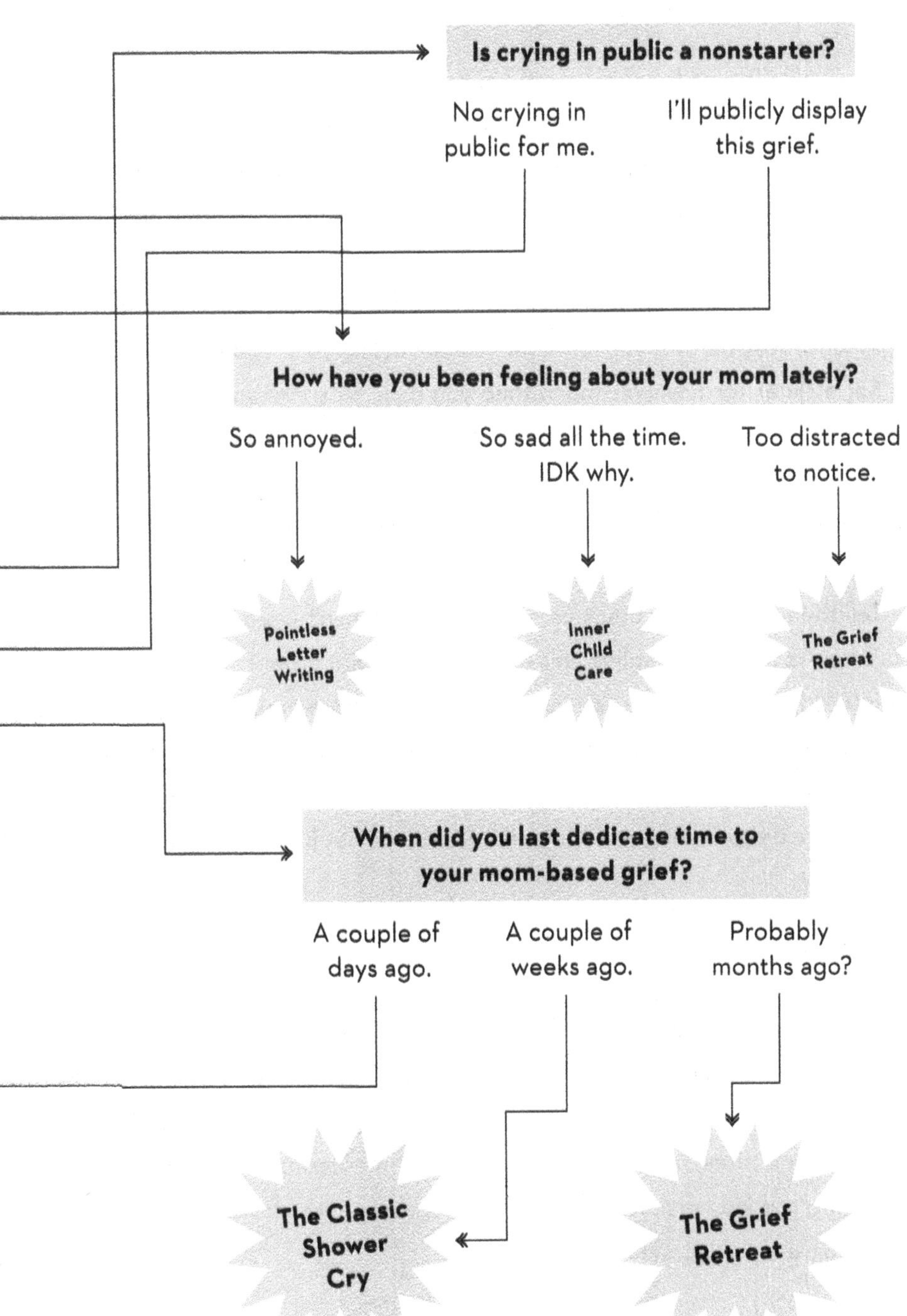

Is crying in public a nonstarter?
No crying in public for me.
I'll publicly display this grief.
How have you been feeling about your mom lately?
So annoyed.
So sad all the time. IDK why.
Too distracted to notice.
Pointless Letter Writing
Inner Child Care
The Grief Retreat
When did you last dedicate time to your mom-based grief?
A couple of days ago.
A couple of weeks ago.
Probably months ago?
The Classic Shower Cry
The Grief Retreat

Pointless Letter Writing

When you're short on time and overwhelmed with chronic sorrow, this can be the easiest way to sit with those feelings and then get on with your day. If you've got a notes app on your phone, an open Word doc on your computer, or paper and pencil handy, you can turn those feelings into words and process what's coming up for you.

Here's how: If you can, find a quiet place. A bathroom stall, your car in the parking lot—wherever you feel comfortable feeling your feelings will do.

Set a timer for however much time you have to spare and take out your writing or typing utensil of choice. Since we're writing a letter here, start by addressing who it may concern. It could be your mom, for sure. It could also be a younger version of yourself, an emotion that's coming up for you ("Dear Anger . . ."), or a fake pen pal.

Tell them everything that's on your mind. It doesn't need to follow a structure. As the name implies, this letter has no point other than getting you into grief mode. Write as much as you can before your timer goes off. When you're done, throw it in the (literal or digital) trash or save it to read to a therapist (or yourself) later. Whatever you do with your pointless letter, take a deep breath, get yourself a treat, and get back to life mode.

Inner-Child Care

Perhaps you've heard of inner-child work. It's a therapy term that usually refers to the practice of acknowledging the parts of you that still feel hurt or unhealed from your childhood, a.k.a. the inner child. The idea is that you can address and repair the impact of messed-up experiences by showing the kid version of you some compassion. It's also sometimes called reparenting yourself.

If your social algorithm isn't already entrenched in these types of ideas, this can sound abstract. Still, picturing your younger self—maybe right after a traumatic incident with your mom—can help you see your experiences (even if they were just last week) from a new perspective. You might realize that the way your mom treated you was unhealthy or even abusive, so it's reasonable that you feel some type of way about her now. Instead of dwelling on that fact, you can mentally care for yourself, providing the attention and affection your caregiver didn't.

Get started: Find a quiet, comfy place where you can close your eyes, or at least soften your gaze and look downward. If you've been ruminating on a specific moment with your mom, let that memory bubble up. If you've been in your chronic sorrow for no apparent reason, think about a painful moment with your mom. It doesn't need to be extreme. Any moment that makes you feel sad, angry, or let down will work. Another option: Picture a photo of yourself as a kid or find the physical (or digital) version.

Once you've got a past version of you in mind, start to interact with them. What do they need or want from Current You in this moment? It could be a hug or someone to tell them what they're going through isn't fair. Perhaps they want to do something fun to feel better after their experience with your mom. Let them express what they want.

Meditate on this for as long as you want or have time for. Thirty minutes could be plenty.

The Classic Shower Cry

When you've got an hour or two till you have to be somewhere, you can multitask by using the getting-ready time as grief time too. This can be helpful if it's been just a little too long since your last grief mode moment. No one wants that shit sneaking up on them.

How to do it: This one is, you know, relatively self-explanatory. Get in the shower, cry, get out, get ready.

Still, I've got some suggestions: Try enticing your grief with a moody or sad playlist. You could also prep for your shower cry by writing down the losses that have been on your mind lately. What have you been ruminating about? What feels hard for you to let go of? Just jotting down a couple of thought starters in a notes app is fine. Then, let it flow. Once the shower is over, it's time to reenter life mode. Well done.

If you decide to cancel your plans, you could follow the same procedure but swap your shower for a sad soak.

The Grief Retreat

To grow from grief, we have to get familiar with swinging back and forth between feeling the loss and living your life. But if you haven't dedicated time to those intense emotions around your relationship with your mom, a little grief retreat could make you more comfortable with chronic sorrow. You know, feel it to heal it and whatnot.

The assignment: Dedicate a day to moving back and forth between grief mode and life mode. Your sadventure can include any or all of the activities I've described. Other useful options might include calling a friend to vent, watching a movie that brings out your grief, or rereading chapters three and four.

Just avoid the urge to wallow. Plan breaks after each grief activity to do fun or neutral activities unrelated to your mom. You could listen to a podcast and bake, go for a walk with a friend, watch a funny movie, take in a basketball game, or get some work and errands done. Whatever helps you move out of grief.

Again, grieving doesn't have to be a drawn-out thing. The goal is to make grief mode a regular part of your life—not a quarterly event. So use this solo retreat to jumpstart a more loss-friendly lifestyle.

Step 4: Find your new normal.

We've entered the *So, now what?* stage of the grieving experience.

After the last few steps, you should have a pretty good idea of what's missing in your relationship with your mom and why those things mean so much to you. From there you can ask, *What do I want*?

Before you answer, a caveat: Sometimes, the things we want aren't possible. We want our moms to see our side. We want them to give more fucks. We want them to be different. None of that is our business, though. You can't turn your mom into a different person.

What you *can* do is change the way you respond to who she is and the circumstances she created. Here's one way this could play out:

Say you and your mom have been arguing about politics since 2020, and you're taken aback by her new opinions (or at least, they're new to you). You grew up thinking of your mom as someone who had a certain set of values, but the opinions she's voiced in the last few years seem completely offtrack. You wonder, *How the hell could she think this way, and when did things change?*

Whenever you hear a political ad on TV or read some headline in your social feed, your mom immediately comes to mind. When spending time with your mom, you're on edge when anything news or politics related comes up. Plus, it's hard to be yourself around her. You're worried the things you say will be thrown back in your face or judged.

In this scenario, you're grieving the loss of shared values and your idea of who your mom was before they started cosigning these views. After dual process model–ing your way through this, you realize your grief is saying, *Hey, I want to have more in common with my mom. I want to understand how they think. I want to be myself around them.*

Now that you see the red flags your grief is throwing, you can do something about it. You can ask yourself, *If this is what it is, how do I want to move forward?*

If you and your mom are otherwise close, you could tell her how her political views make you feel and how they're impacting your relationship. You can explain that you feel distanced from her. Maybe you can find new things in common so the political differences don't seem as major. Or, you could ask questions to genuinely understand her stance—even if you don't agree. You could also manage the situation on your own by avoiding political talk and creating an escape plan for when it comes up.

Every experience of navigating mom-related grief is going to be different, of course. Still, paying attention to the losses that activate your grief and pausing to consider what you can realistically do about them is how you give your grief what it wants. You're finding ways to work within your current reality, losses and all.

Step 5: Redefine your identity.

Let me say it louder for the people in the back: Grieving means adapting to a world that's different from the one you thought you were living in or thought you *should be* living in. That can impact how you see yourself.

When you accept that your mom isn't who you want her to be, you're saying goodbye to an idealized version of your past, present, *and* future. You're giving up the glossy way you described your childhood, the fantasy of what holidays and birthdays will look like as you get older, or how your mom will show up as a grandparent for your kids. And letting go of those idealistic visions means losing a part of your own identity, writes Dr. Roos in *Non-Death Loss and Grief.*

Like Step 4, Step 5 entails deciding what you want to do with your reality. If your mom is going to be like this for the foreseeable future, who do *you* want to be? Ditching the fantasy means redefining yourself.

Could you be a person who isn't that close with your mom? Could you be someone who doesn't worry about what your mom thinks of your job, haircut, or partner, or one who dares to block their mom's number?

Here's my identity these days: I am someone who sees my mom at holidays and family events. On my wedding day, I asked my friends to button the back of my dress while blasting "We Will Rock You" instead of hoping my mom would volunteer for this traditionally emotional moment. I'm a recovering golden child who's OK with being the villain in (untrue) family gossip. I'm good!

Step 6: Create a coping plan.

The grief may never go away, but we can build ourselves a little safety net made of internal and external resources to manage it, write Dr. Harris and Dr. Winokuer in "Living Losses."

To locate the resources nearest you, think about the most activating (see: triggering) moments, then ask: What can you do to make them more bearable? Who or what else can help?

Say Mother's Day is notoriously tough on you. The Instagram captions, the brunch plans, the ads celebrating "the person who has always been there for you."

So, on the second Sunday in May, can you decide to stay in bed, order a bagel, and watch horror movies all day? Sure can! Or maybe you call up someone who gets your situation to vent about how bad it is. You might cry in the shower and then go about your Sunday as usual. You could also make an effort to celebrate the other caregivers in your life (including yourself, if that's applicable).

Thinking ahead, planning for the big feelings, and taking care of yourself is the best way to deal with the grief you know is headed your way.

YOUR REGULAR REMINDER: THERAPY COULD BE HELPFUL!

Maybe you didn't seriously consider hiring a therapist back when we first talked about doing that in chapter seven. I get it. But when I asked Dr. Neimeyer how to tell if you need a therapist to get you through grief, he basically said that if you're reading this book, you could probably use a therapist. I don't think he's wrong, but in case you're still not sold, here are some other guidelines from him: If you've been stuck in the same cycles for months or years, therapy could be useful. Same goes if you feel so overwhelmed that you're acting in ways that could hurt yourself or others. When in doubt, it's worth giving it a shot!

AM I HEALED YET?

OK, you already know the answer to that question is no. Neither you nor I will ever be fully healed, or done grieving, no matter how much we do it. That's the fun part of chronic sorrow. But it does get easier! When you incorporate your loss into the story of your life and your understanding of the world, navigating triggers gets more chill. The usual suspects might not even faze you anymore.

To measure advancement on thy healing journey/growth trajectory/emotional advancement, Dr. Neimeyer and his colleagues created a questionnaire called the Integration of Stressful Life Experiences Scale.* I've adapted it here as a quiz for gauging our mom-based losses.

Instructions

For each of the following statements, circle the number that aligns with your perspective right now. When you're done, add up the numbers and divide them by 16. The higher the number, the "greater the integration," write the authors. That's a good thing, because remixing loss into your life is the whole point of grief.

You can take this quiz every few weeks or months to track how it's going. It's OK if you're up one week and down another. Shit happens.

1. **Because of my relationship with my mom, the world seems like a confusing and scary place.**

   strongly agree 1 2 3 4 5 strongly disagree

2. **I have made sense of my relationship with my mom.**

   strongly agree 5 4 3 2 1 strongly disagree

3. **If or when I talk about my relationship with my mom, I believe people see me differently.**

   strongly agree 1 2 3 4 5 strongly disagree

* Developed by Jason M. Holland, Joseph Currier, Rachel A. Coleman, and Robert A. Neimeyer, and published in 2010 in the *International Journal of Stress Management*.

4. **I have difficulty integrating my relationship with my mom into my understanding of the world.**

   strongly agree 1 2 3 4 5 strongly disagree

5. **Because of my relationship with my mom, I feel like I'm in a crisis of faith.**

   strongly agree 1 2 3 4 5 strongly disagree

6. **My relationship with my mom is incomprehensible to me.**

   strongly agree 1 2 3 4 5 strongly disagree

7. **My goals and hopes for the future don't make sense because of my relationship with my mom.**

   strongly agree 1 2 3 4 5 strongly disagree

8. **I am perplexed by my relationship with my mom.**

   strongly agree 1 2 3 4 5 strongly disagree

9. **Because of my relationship with my mom, I don't know where to go next in my life.**

   strongly agree 1 2 3 4 5 strongly disagree

10. **I would have an easier time talking about my life if I left my relationship with my mom out.**

    strongly agree 1 2 3 4 5 strongly disagree

11. **My beliefs and values are less clear because of my relationship with my mom.**

    strongly agree 1 2 3 4 5 strongly disagree

12. **I don't understand myself because of my relationship with my mom.**

    strongly agree 1 2 3 4 5 strongly disagree

13. **Because of my relationship with my mom, I have a harder time feeling like I'm part of something larger than myself.**

    strongly agree 1 2 3 4 5 strongly disagree

14. **My relationship with my mom has made me feel less purposeful.**

    strongly agree 1 2 3 4 5 strongly disagree

15. **I haven't been able to put the pieces of my life together because of my relationship with my mom.**

    strongly agree 1 2 3 4 5 strongly disagree

16. **Because of my relationship with my mom, life seems more random.**

    strongly agree 1 2 3 4 5 strongly disagree

TOTAL SCORE ____ DIVIDED BY 16 = ____

Results

If your score (the total of your numbers divided by 16) is less than 3: You're likely in the thick of it right now, and nothing makes sense. Like a GPS from 2008, your brain is still recalculating its way out of a grief hole—there's some lag time.

While it's not fun, you're doing what has to be done to find your way through this: reconciling what you hoped for in a mom with who your mom really is. Making your relationship fit into the story of your life is grueling work. Some days (or weeks, or months, or years) are just harder than others.

The more you can validate your loss and make time for your feelings, the closer you'll get to redefining your identity and the meaning of this loss for your life. You didn't choose this relationship, but you get to decide what to do with it. That's how you get to acceptance, the closest healing dupe there is.

If you scored a 3 or higher: This is what progress feels like, friend. You're doing what grief researchers call meaning-making, or making sense of a loss, write Dr. Neimeyer and Krawchuck in *Non-Death Loss and Grief*. With a higher score like yours, you're likely more comfortable with validating your losses, feeling your grief, and rethinking who you want to be in light of that. That's how you make sense of this relationship (or nonrelationship) with your mom.

With time, you might even find purpose in this loss and how it shaped you (if you haven't already!). Maybe this unhealthy relationship with your mom made you more empathetic, or the adversity helped you develop skills you wouldn't have otherwise. Maybe it just is what it is and that's all the meaning you need. That's fine too.

CHAPTER 9

Dealing with Your Mom

You felt your feelings and cried to a bespoke playlist that hit you right where it hurts. You pendulated your way from grief to being normal and back to grief again like Miley Cyrus on a wrecking ball.

You emerge fresh, emotionally exfoliated. You feel moderately fine with the fact that your mom will, for example, never act her emotional age. You start considering what life would be like if you spent less time worrying about her thoughts and feelings (or maybe you finally experience that). Your new and improved grief now comes with 20 percent *less* rumination.

But then your mom calls, and you're back in the thick of it.

Dealing with your mom while trying to heal is a next-level challenge. That said, now that you have a better understanding of your feelings and what you've lost, it can be easier to manage this relationship.

In this chapter, I'll give you a little primer on the best practices for interacting with your mom as you're going through the grieving process (or anytime, really).

Should you tell your mom how you feel about your relationship and the ways she's hurt you? When is that helpful, and how do you do it? I got you.

You'll also learn how to talk to her about your feelings by considering how she's responded to that in the past. And then I've got some very specific strategies for confronting your mom about your relationship, depending on your comfort level.

Much to discuss!

STEP 1: CONSIDER HOW YOUR MOM RESPONDS TO FEEDBACK.

You've likely spent a lifetime trying to express your needs to your mom in one way or another. Since you're here reading this, I suspect those attempts were largely unsuccessful.

Whether they failed because your mom is emotionally immature, has a mental health condition, or some other factor, you've probably learned that she isn't a safe place to put your feelings, says Whitney Goodman, creator of the Calling Home community. That intel can help you determine the best way to engage with her now.

Think about the last time you tried to tell your mom how her behavior made you feel. Whether it was last week or twenty years ago, what was her reaction? Did she burst into tears and wait for you to comfort her? Did she blow you off or belittle you? Did she respond as if you're out to get her?

Then, ponder this: Is there a larger pattern going on here? Is this her typical response when confronted? Consider how she reacts when other people tell her about herself. Is she defensive or receptive to that feedback? Maybe it's a mix of both.

You can also consult people who know your mom well. Have they noticed the way your mom handles this kind of thing? Is Mom's reaction predictable?

Whatever the case, your mom's default response to criticism, especially when it's coming from you, will likely be the same now as it's always been. "You can only meet someone as far as they'll go," says Goodman.

STEP 2: USE THOSE OBSERVATIONS TO DETERMINE HOW YOU TALK TO THEM (OR DON'T).

Of course, your mom may be open to constructive criticism about your relationship. That's totally possible! If this is true for you, that's a big green flag to let it all out so your mom can make it right.

For everyone else, figuring out the best way to communicate—or whether to do it at all—is more complicated. There's no perfect formula for telling your mom how she's hurt you and how you feel about it. For some relationships, it doesn't matter how strategically you frame your feedback. Those moms aren't able or willing to hear it.

That's why Goodman recommends using the data points you've collected to strategize how to address the problem. Here are a couple of options.

If you know she'll take your feedback as an insult...

Say your mom is notoriously defensive when presented with opportunities for growth. They're like this with you, your siblings, their boss, and anyone else who dares to confront them.

Whatever you do, do not tell an emotionally immature person or someone with narcissistic tendencies that they're emotionally immature or have narcissistic tendencies. Even if those things are true, it will not go well, says Goodman.

In this case, you'll need to sit with the fact that explaining how her actions made you feel will not elicit a response like "You're so right! Here's how I'm going to change that." If that truth still hurts, it might be helpful to do a little grief work around that loss (I refer you to chapter eight).

With your expectations reset, consider what interactions feel productive. If you know your mom won't hear you, let alone change her ways, it might not make sense to share your grievances with her. Instead, you might decide it's more feasible to change *your* behavior. You can start living in a way that's aligned with how you feel. You could set limits around the time you spend together or what you talk about. Do you want to keep these limits in place until you hit a new level of acceptance? Could you stick to them for the foreseeable future? If you're already doing this, would it be helpful to further restrict contact with your mom? It's totally your call. (By the way, this is called *setting boundaries*. More on boundaries in chapter ten.)

The thing about setting limits, pulling back, and going against the grain is that your mom will probably notice. She may even be upset that you're not catering to her the way you used to. When that happens, your assignment is to get comfortable disappointing your mom, says Goodman.

She adds that you don't have to give your mom a big speech about why you're not answering her calls during the workday or why you're not coming home for the holidays. That probably wouldn't help her understand anyway. Instead, you can deal with your mom's pushback on a case-by-case basis. Text her that you can't talk right now. Tell her it's easier for you to hang back this holiday season. Or don't say anything at all. The hardest part of all this is learning to be content when she's not. The more work you do on your own, the easier it gets.

If you're not sure how she'll react or you want to give her the benefit of the doubt...

Sometimes you need more information before making changes. Even if your mom is emotionally immature, hasn't been receptive to your feelings in the past, or both, you could feel compelled to give her another chance. That's fair! Maybe, like me, you felt like you were in a one-sided fight. I reasoned that if my mom didn't know there was a problem, she didn't have a chance to fix it.

Alternatively, you might want to let it rip after years of putting up with garbage behavior. That's cool and understandable as well.

Still, in any of these cases, it's unhelpful to tell your mom that, for example, she's a narcissist who needs therapy. But you can give her feedback on how her behavior impacts you, says Goodman.

Leaving the mental health language out of it, you can use the confrontation sandwich method:

1. Tell her why you're giving her feedback. Ideally, this is a positive reason, like you want a better relationship, you want to give her a chance to make things right, and you want family time to feel less tense. All good things.
2. Chase that positivity with your critique. For your own safety and the safety of those around you (kidding, but really . . .), use "I" statements. That sounds like: "When you ________, I feel (or think) ________ because ________."
3. Explain what you'd like to do moving forward and restate the positive reason for that.

If she takes ownership of her behavior ("I'm sorry you feel that way" and "I didn't mean to" deflect accountability and therefore don't count), that's a step in the right direction. She should also say what she'll do differently in the future. If she's not clear on what that will be, you can ask her.

On the other hand, if she tries to manipulate you by making excuses, getting passive-aggressive, overreacting, downplaying your emotions, or making fun of you, well, that's useful data.

Also, beware of appeasement. If your mom just wants to get this conversation done with, she might try to smooth things over and change the subject. So don't be afraid to challenge any HR-worthy answers.

Then, put what you've learned in your mental spreadsheet and let it guide your interactions going forward, says Goodman.

STEP 3: TAKE CARE OF YOURSELF.

After working on steps 1 and 2, you'll need to get yourself out of grief mode and into life mode. You know the drill here. Schedule something delightful, like getting ice cream or hugging a dog. Then, because the dual process model demands it, you can (and should) come back to your feelings about this interaction when you've got the time and space to do it.

Do not underestimate how much care you might need after confronting your mom or your relationship with her. It is really fucking hard.

THREE MORE WAYS TO CONFRONT YOUR MOM

We discussed the confrontation sandwich method, a tried-and-true form of being assertive in any situation. But there are many more options for telling your mom what's up.

Obviously, the best strategy for you hinges on how comfortable you feel doing it and your goal. While you may never feel great talking to your mom about your childhood trauma, you can make it less anxiety inducing.

Here are a few options I've curated based on my experience with my mom and as a mental health editor and reporter.

The State of the Relationship Speech

Confrontation level: Novice

What it is: A rebuttal-resistant form of interaction that minimizes opportunity for defensiveness and manipulation. The goal here is to say everything you want to say in your mom's presence. Plus, you'll allot some time for questions at the end. It's like a corporate all-hands for your relationship: It's not a discussion, it's an announcement.

Who it's for: Anyone who struggles to open up to their mom, has received plenty of "Sorry you feel that way"-adjacent responses in the past, and knows their mom won't change. I also recommend it for those who can't stop the mental arguments playing out in their heads. Saying what you need to say can stop the madness.

How to do it: As with any speech, prepare ahead of time. But don't stress too hard—a list of bullet points is plenty. While you can structure your speech any way you like, it might help to start by briefly explaining why you're about to break down the state of your relationship. Does your mom expect all the perks of a close mother-child relationship without doing any of the emotional work? Do you feel you have an unhealthy dynamic? Do you want her to know what kinds of interactions hurt you? Have you talked about her behavior before, but she refused to change? Tell her why we are all gathered here today before really getting into it.

Then, explain what this relationship is like from your point of view. You can refer back to your childhood or name recent issues to make your point. I'm a fan of doing both. Once you've listed how you feel about your relationship and the examples that support your perspective, you can restate why you're making this announcement. Things like "I need to tell you how I feel," "I need space to think about how to move forward," or "I'm not OK with this dynamic" are great reasons.

Last but not least, make space for your mom's questions or reaction by asking, literally, "Do you have any questions?" This makes it clear you're not looking for a rebuttal; you're seeking to clarify what you've already said.

The Classic Q&A

Confrontation level: Intermediate

What it is: An exchange of questions (from you) and answers (from your mom). This interaction can help you name the problem by digging deeper into why it's happening and how to fix it.

Who it's for: If you rarely second-guess your experience with your mom or your feelings about her, you're OK with some back and forth, and you want to hear her out, this one is for you. If your mom is prone to manipulative behavior, it's not.

How to do it: At the top of the conversation, explain the goal. That could sound like "I've been hurt and confused by some of your behavior, and I'd like to ask you some questions about it." But you don't have to be that specific; you can just say, "Hey, do you have time to talk through some things I've noticed about our relationship?" She might not be excited, but hopefully she's willing to engage meaningfully.

From there, start going through your questions. After each one, make sure you give your mom the opportunity to share her perspective. This can be nerve-racking, so writing your Qs beforehand can help you stay on track.

As she explains her side, try to listen closely. Avoid thinking about the next question or your retort. (If you're nervous, record the conversation or take notes so you can review it in a better headspace.)

When you're finished, you can ask if she has questions or tell her that you'll circle back with some thoughts on her response. Take all the time you need to assess how it went and what you want to do with your learnings.

Pointing Out the Problem in Real Time

Confrontation level: Advanced

What it is: Calling out bad behavior as it happens. It's a super-helpful way to make your mom aware in the moment of the hurtful things she says or does and how you'd prefer she treat you.

Who it's for: If you talk to your mom often and you're relatively comfortable being honest about your feelings, this might be a fit. Those who are (understandably) stuck in their conflict-averse ways should try something less intense.

How to do it: When your mom does something that makes you feel bad, tell her right away.

For example, if you two are catching up over coffee and, out of nowhere, your mom throws a verbal dagger like "I'm not surprised you're still single," that's your cue to speak up.

If you're someplace where this kind of back-and-forth is less appropriate, like a family BBQ or a baby's baptism (it could happen), wait till you get home and then bring it up. But the less time between the hurtful thing occurring and your response to it, the better.

To be real, addressing the issues as they happen doesn't mean your mom will actually understand your perspective or change. She might even ignore you. That said, this (like the other methods) is still a solid way to gather intel on how she responds to your feelings. If she consistently ignores you or makes excuses, set some limits to protect yourself.

HOW I DEALT WITH MY MOM: A CASE STUDY

Not long after starting therapy, my mom and nana came to visit me in New York City.

I came home after a long, try-hard day at work, bearing bagels and schmear for the weekend. I opened the door to my studio apartment where all four of us (including my now-husband Sean) were staying. I said something like "YAY! You're here! I got bagels for tomorrow morning!"

Without skipping a beat, Foxy deadpanned, "What about dinner? We're hungry." This was the first time I'd seen her in six months.

Over the course of that visit, Foxy engaged in more conversations with strangers than with my nana and me. She ate grapes and threw the stems on my apartment floor ("Where am I supposed to put them?"). She offered to pay for dinner a total of zero times. On her way home, she called to say how much fun she had seeing the sights.

This list of grievances could come off as petty. When you zoom out, though, these are all examples of a larger pattern. My bagels, the happenings in my life she didn't ask about, and my floor apparently weren't important to her. It hurt to have that fact waved in my face as we shared five hundred square feet for five days.

So my therapist encouraged me to tell her how mad I was.

I'd never explicitly told Foxy how she'd hurt me before. My tactic was to ignore or laugh off as much as possible. When I couldn't, I'd correct her behavior: "Stop ditching us to talk to random people! Please wear a bra while we're all sleeping in the same room! Throw your trash in the garbage!" Then she'd scoff and say I was always criticizing her. This routine was embedded in the DNA of our relationship.

When I called to air my grievances, I tried to stay calm, explaining why future visits would be capped at four days or less. I brought up the bagel thing, the bra thing, and the grape thing. She scoffed. I lost it.

Twenty years of pent-up emotions came raging out. I told her how it seemed like she doesn't give a shit about me, my feelings, or spending time with me. I told her that every time she leaves me and whoever we're with to chat with strangers, it hurts. I told her I don't care if she talks to randos at coffee shops; I do care that she doesn't give me the same time and attention.

I said the core of this whole issue is that I want my mom to *want* to hang out with me. I wanted my mom. Period. As I explained all that, I was sobbing and yelling in a way I'd never done with her before. I think she was caught off guard.

She said she was sorry I was so upset, and she didn't mean to make me feel this bad. I sensed she didn't get it. She changed the subject, and I let her.

I'd expressed myself explicitly. She didn't take the bait to repair the situation. Thus, I had confirmation that any future conversations in which I shared my feelings would be futile.

Over the next five years, I started to pull away. We spoke every three weeks, then once a month, then every other month. I limited how much I shared with her about my life: "Everything is fine. Work is busy. Sean is good."

Foxy noticed. Whenever we spoke, she'd remind me that I wasn't answering my phone or telling her the things I told the rest of my family.

I'd complain to my therapist about the guilt trips and manipulative texts, and how sick I was of thinking about her all the time and worrying what she'd say to the rest of my family.

My therapist always asked, "Why don't you say that you're pulling back because she isn't nice to you?" I reasoned that it would be pointless, since nothing changed after the last time I confronted her. Plus, I got really caught up trying to predict her response and plan a rebuttal. Each of those mental arguments ended with me deciding to do nothing.

Then, my therapist said, "What if the point of telling your mom about how you see your relationship isn't to change her? What if it's for you to say how you feel and what you want? Throw the ball back in her court."

So I crafted my State of the Relationship Speech, read it to her over the phone, and took detailed notes on her response. I emailed the speech to her later so she could refer to it as needed.

Those brutally honest chats helped me grow in ways my conflict-averse, Libra-rising ass could never have seen coming.

LESSONS LEARNED

No one has more knowledge about your relationship with your mom than you. Yet, despite decades of information gathering, sometimes we need more details before we can fully grasp the reality of this dynamic. And now you know how reflecting on past interactions or confronting your mom could help you do that. With examples at the ready of how she treats you and responds to your feedback, you'll find it easier to see your relationship as it currently stands. That can help you scooch a little closer to acceptance.

Whether or not you need a conversation with your mom to get clear on the health of your relationship, what you learn from that conversation can help you set more effective boundaries. And that's what we're about to do next.

CHAPTER 10

How to Set Boundaries

I truly sucked at the whole boundary-setting process. I'd spent most of my life working around my mom's behavior. I knew how she'd react to any given interaction with me, and I tried to be as compliant as possible. I also did the emotional heavy lifting to maintain our relationship. I felt it was up to me to present information about my life, find moments of connection, and listen to Foxy vent.

I kept that up through my early thirties. I'd call every week. Sometimes I'd multitask and call her while I was running errands so she could go off in my ear while I bought toilet paper.

I put my need for emotional depth aside to accommodate how she wanted to show up in the relationship. If I did the work, then I could pretend we were close, or at least close-ish.

I was also quick to sacrifice my time and energy for connection. Maybe *this* time, applying her eyeliner would transform her indifference into appreciation. Instead, it felt as if she were a teenager tolerating my efforts to get closer. I'm such a helicopter daughter.

But once I became aware of how much work it took to maintain a relationship that didn't feel good, it was harder to keep up. I answered the phone, but her twenty-minute monologue hurt more than before. Thanks, therapy.

Even a month after I made my State of the Relationship Speech, declaring how I felt and the ways she hurt me, nothing changed. The most significant effort she made happened when I called to say happy Easter. It was the first time we'd spoken since my big speech. When she finished talking about her plans, she asked, "Is there anything you'd like me to ask you, you know, to be a good mom?"

I didn't have the capacity to keep coaching, so I just said, "No."

Despite the jarring clarity about where we stood, I just couldn't bring myself to set firmer boundaries. I believed my mom had the same emotional needs that I did. I would be crushed if she stopped answering my calls or said she could only talk once a month. I didn't want to hurt her. But then my therapist asked, "What if it's not that deep for her? What if she isn't hurt that you're not answering or worried that you don't care about her? What if she's just mad because she can't access you?"

Damn.

That theory made sense to me, though. In all of the times my mom guilt-tripped me for not being in touch, she never said, "Did I do something wrong? I miss how much we used to talk. I miss *you*." Instead, she sent passive-aggressive texts or complained to other people.

Even with that revelation, my boundary-setting trajectory was not up and to the right. I'd make some progress, then feel bad and go back to my old ways. Then, when a friend suggested blocking my mom's number, something I'd never considered before, it clicked. Throughout my life, I treated my mom the way I wanted to be treated, not the way she treated me. But it turns out the golden rule has fine print I missed: You don't have to make an effort for people who don't do the same for you—even if that person is your mom.

I thought about blocking her for a while and finally decided to go for it—with caveats. I would unblock her for holidays, birthdays, and anniversaries. I wasn't cutting her off; I was taking space.

I hoped blocking Foxy would get her out of my head while also allowing for contact on occasions when I wanted to hear from her or show that I cared about her. I *thought* that would be enough for me to stop dwelling on her thoughts and feelings.

But when I unblocked her on my birthday, it did not go as I planned. She texted me: *Happy Birthday * sunglasses emoji * Call me if you want to talk. You NEVER answer when I call *weary face emoji* If your dr told you to do this so be it *rainbow emoji**

Despite the confusing use of emoji and aggressive passive aggression, I did call her. Over the phone, she wished me a happy birthday and then went on about where she was, what she did that week, the class she took at the YMCA, the cat, and how she's looking for a new job—the usual. I hung up and blocked her . . . only to unblock her a few days later to say thanks for the birthday card. It contained a coupon for 20 percent off at Express.

Yep, boundaries are fucking hard. When you spend a majority of your life prioritizing your mom's needs and feelings over yours, it's easy to forget you don't have to. You can choose to do what's best for you.

That's what we're here to learn.

So, let's look at how to put yourself first—even when it's uncomfortable—by creating healthy, flexible boundaries with your mom.

We'll explore what boundaries are, how they work, when they don't, and how to put them in place. Then, I've got an exercise to help you brainstorm your ideal boundaries and get them from your brain to your mom's with minimal drama.

WHAT BOUNDARIES ARE AND WHY WE NEED THEM

If it feels like your social feeds are obsessed with boundaries lately, you're not wrong. Therapists, lifestyle influencers, and that friend from college who recently discovered meditation and Mel Robbins are all about a well-boundaried life. However, like "healing," the definition of a boundary isn't that obvious. Maybe that's why so many people misuse it.

Generally speaking, boundaries are a physical or mental line in the sand that separates us from other people, says clinical psychologist and *Permission to Come Home* author Dr. Jenny Tzu-Mei Wang. Within relationships, boundaries lay out how we'd like to be treated. They define what we're willing to put up with and what we're not. When you set these limits, you can stay true to your thoughts, emotions, and individuality while coexisting with others. Love to see that.

Though "boundaries" sounds bouncer-like—and they can be used that way, keeping unhealthy dynamics out of your life—they can also be more like school crossing guards, keeping you safe while allowing for healthy interactions.

Here's what boundaries can look like in real life:

* Not answering the phone after 9 PM
* Not discussing politics at family events
* Not venting about your partner to your mom
* Not lending your mom more than $20 at a time
* Skipping out on hugs if they make you uncomfortable

Setting boundaries isn't just about avoiding things, though. Boundaries can also include actionable expectations for your relationship like emotionally mature communication (especially during conflict). You might also create boundaries that maintain your individuality, like being open about your opinions or parts of your identity. Designating and protecting quality time count too.

Sometimes boundaries are things you say out loud, and sometimes they're not. For example, by avoiding certain people (like your mom) or situations (like being at your mom's house), you can enact your boundaries without telling anyone, says Dr. Wang.

Of course, you can also express, enact, or enforce your boundaries with others by using your words:

"I'm not going to read those weird chain emails you keep sending me."
"I won't pretend everything's fine when it's not."
"I'm not going to respond to your texts right away, especially if you send forty-two in a row."

In the end, boundaries can be whatever you want them to be, as long as they establish a sense of self and safety within your relationships.

Here are just a few of their extremely lucrative perks when navigating an unhealthy dynamic with your mom.

Boundaries protect our individuality.

Not to get existential on you, but boundaries give us permission to have an identity, thoughts, emotions, and behaviors that differ from others'. When you decide not to engage with a person or their behavior, or say, "I don't agree and here's why," you're being true to you.

Even in the best mother–child relationships, boundaries help you exist as an independent adult. Setting some parameters can minimize their input on your life, enable self-discovery, and provide a little privacy—all while maintaining a relationship that feels good. Hell yeah.

Individuation—a fancy word that describes the process of figuring out who you are, distinct from everyone else—can be really challenging in the context of your mom. As you know, we are born to be our mom's biggest fan. That means separating our preferences, beliefs, and actions from theirs isn't always easy.

For example, if you say that you really don't love the salad bar at Ruby Tuesday, their personal fave in this scenario, and they respond as if you've punched them in the face—you're not likely to do that again.

Likewise, not adhering to your mom's preferred religion, career path, or political take can result in eyerolls, verbal assault, or perhaps the silent treatment. And because we just want our moms to love and approve of us, even the quietest yuck to our yum can sting.

Said sting could have you responding in a lot of different ways. You might rebel, going further in the opposite direction. ("You heard me, Ruby Tuesday is a scam!") On the other end, you might decide your thoughts and opinions don't matter or that expressing them to your mom is more trouble than it's worth.

Dr. Wang says that many people who avoid setting boundaries with their mom wind up unsure of what they like and don't. Your mom has more power in this dynamic, so the line between the two of you can get blurry, she explains: "Often the more dominant personality will subsume the more passive one, and we can kind of become one."

Boundaries help us find ourselves and maintain that individuality, even when we face backlash. In dysfunctional relationships with our moms, that's a skill a lot of us could probably strengthen.

Boundaries protect our emotions.

Setting limits can help you care for yourself in any relationship. But with your mom, boundaries are particularly good at defending against triggers.

Our moms know what sets us off, what makes us do what they want, and how we'll respond to many a situation. And with great power comes great potential for abuse (that's how that line goes, right?).

As kids, we often find ways to work around caregivers who use this knowledge against us, like avoiding certain topics, keeping opinions to ourselves, or shifting how we act around them. These maneuvers help us stay connected to the people we rely on most to meet our basic needs. Ugh, attachment.

As adults, though, we have the opportunity to rework that unhealthy, painful relationship so it functions better for us. We get to say, "You know what, this makes me feel pretty terrible. I'm going to see myself out."

Armed with a solid set of boundaries, you can engage with your mom in a way that doesn't desert your emotional needs. You can leave when she says something hurtful, you can share your perspective instead of holding back, or you can reassure yourself that you deserve to be treated with empathy and respect.

Boundaries protect our resources.

In addition to keeping your identity and feelings safe and sound, setting limits can safeguard your time, energy, and money.

When we let moms walk all over us, whether they know they're doing it or not, we're more likely to feel depleted and burned out. That leaves us with less energy for our lives outside this relationship, says Dr. Wang.

You might be distracted at work, spend most of your date nights venting about your mom, or feel too tired to go out with your friends. You might even delay paying bills because your mom guilted you into buying her a new washing machine. None of that is OK.

I cordially invite you to preserve your energy by choosing what they can and can't take from you. Ultimately, says Dr. Wang, you get to choose where your time, attention, and other resources go.

Boundaries protect our relationships.

Even if your mom sucks sometimes, your relationship with her might have some good moments. With emotional guardrails like boundaries, it may be possible to keep the good and lose the bad.

Can't talk about the news without mom delving into their conspiracy theories? Boundary it! Don't want another lecture about going to church? Boundary it!

Because boundaries teach others how you want to be treated, they help you get along with people who don't always make you feel good, says Dr. Wang. Assuming the other person is willing to go along with your new filtration system, boundaries allow you to spend time with them within the safe parts of your relationship.

For example, say you and your mom love to gab about true crime, home decor, and your love life. Yet, you start to lose the plot when she inevitably brings up the fact that you don't attend their house of worship. All hope is not lost! By telling your mom that you're not a church person and you don't want to talk about it anymore, you keep your time together safe.

If you want to stay in touch with your mom, especially while grieving, boundaries are an extremely helpful tool. That's especially true if your mom isn't doing anything to heal up or develop emotionally mature habits, adds Minaa B., therapist and author of *Owning Our Struggles*. Boundaries enable you to work around your mom's emotional immaturity without tolerating any mistreatment.

In the end, you may not have to choose between putting up with hurtful behavior or completely cutting your mom off, Minaa B. explains. "There is a gray area, and you can figure out what that looks like for you to feel safe."

WHAT CAN'T BOUNDARIES DO?

This may sound like sponsored content on behalf of Boundary Co., but there are many things this self-protective measure won't help with.

Boundaries can't be used as a way to punish your mom (or at least they shouldn't).

When you use a boundary to punish your mom, the boundary becomes more about getting a reaction from her than protecting you. "It pulls you back into the dynamic and it can keep you in a cycle of conflict," says Dr. Wang. That's why (in my words, not Dr. Wang's) using a boundary to punish your mom is an abuse of boundary power, according to boundary law.

Boundaries won't change your mom.

Sure, setting a boundary and asking your mom to respect it can shift how they show up in your relationship. But that's not something you should count on. Boundaries are about you and what you're willing to put up with. They're meant to protect you, not train other people to be better.

Boundaries won't get them to see your side.

If your mom hasn't been open to your perspective, feelings, and concerns up to now, chances are she won't start anytime soon. Using boundaries can help you two coexist despite your differences, though. And here's more good news: Your mom doesn't have to get why you're putting this boundary in place for the boundary to work.

WHY DOES SETTING BOUNDARIES FEEL SO HARD?

Even if you're fully subscribed to the boundary narrative, and you know what boundaries can and can't do, the *act* of setting boundaries remains challenging. The reasons behind this are, obviously, extremely nuanced. That said, there are some common reasons why people struggle to stand up for themselves in their relationship with their mom.

Being vulnerable is scary.

Putting yourself out there by saying, "Here's what I need in this relationship and how I would like to be treated," is an act of vulnerability, says Dr. Wang. When you don't go with the other person's flow, they can disagree, do what they want anyway, or even end your relationship. All of those things are forms of rejection, and rejection is not fun.

If you're not used to being vulnerable with your mom, or it's gone badly when you've done it in the past, starting now is a big deal. "Setting boundaries with people who aren't safe or those you've never set limits with before can activate your fight-or-flight response," explains Dr. Wang. "You might feel scared, overwhelmed, or panicky because you're terrified of their reaction."

You're used to being steamrolled.

It's possible your mom low-key (or high-key) trained you to let her do whatever she wants within your relationship. Being praised for people pleasing (or punished for not doing so) can socialize you to forgo boundaries, says Dr. Wang.

Over time, those experiences enforce the idea that you're undeserving of limits and preferences, she adds. If your perspective doesn't matter, why bother speaking up? Compliance can feel like your safest option. Dr. Wang explains that this mindset weakens your ability to express your wants and needs within that relationship (and in general, to be honest).

You think setting boundaries is mean.

For better or worse, people want to be loved and to belong, says Dr. Wang. Those of us who haven't done much boundary-ing can find that creating limits feels like preventing people from loving or accepting us. It can feel like we're cutting people off.

When you and your mom have no guardrails on your interactions, you might assume creating new boundaries is rude or disrespectful. You might even think it will inhibit how close you are or could become.

Same goes if you suspect that mom only loves you when you let her act however she wants. You might think, "Well, if I'm unlovable, then I want to do everything I can to keep her happy," says Dr. Wang. When you nix your boundaries to receive care and attention from your mom, it might keep the peace or even feel good in the short term. But doing that can put you in compromising situations later on.

While those feelings are valid, allowing anyone—including your mom—to mistreat you is ultimately disrespecting yourself. Every type of relationship needs boundaries, says Dr. Wang.

SIGNS YOU NEED BOUNDARIES WITH YOUR MOM

Literally anyone with a mom needs boundaries with them. Still, there are some indicators you *really* need to set parameters with yours. If you can relate to any of the following scenarios, chances are your boundaries could use a little bulking up. Let's assess.

Your mom's behavior sparks Big Feelings.

People do annoying things all the time, but when those people are your mom, and the things she's doing make you feel enraged, depressed, exhausted, or any extreme type of way, that's a red flag.

Dr. Wang says that when we need stronger boundaries with someone, even their everyday actions can trigger a strong emotional response in us. Perhaps you recall my breakdown after an uneventful phone call with my mom. Oftentimes, our feelings can be disproportional to whatever the other person did.

The same shit keeps happening.

Sometimes our emotional response isn't XXL. When your mom keeps doing a thing you don't like, you might feel rightfully upset and confused about why it keeps happening, says Dr. Wang.

This doesn't necessarily mean your mom is doing exactly the same thing over and over again, though it could. Sometimes it's just that a clear theme emerges from her behavior.

Let's say your mom always buys you gifts that seem meant for somebody else: gift cards to stores you don't go to, supplies for a hobby you don't have, or something else that just feels really impersonal. If that's the whole story, it might not be that big of a deal. But if they're also oblivious to other basic details of your life, it means you're constantly reminded your mom doesn't listen to you or care about who you are as an individual.

The uncomfortable feelings tend to linger.

Even if you're used to your mom's usual tricks and know why they're this way, your emotional reaction to whatever they said or did (or didn't say or do) can linger, says Dr. Wang.

You might keep the feelings to yourself, where they just weigh on you indefinitely. Or you might transfer them to another area of your life, like your kids, your partner, a coworker, or the person ahead of you at the ATM. If this sounds familiar, consider this your sign to think, *Hmm, maybe I need some boundaries.*

HOW TO SET A HEALTHY BOUNDARY

When I gave my State of the Relationship Speech to my mom, I ended the call saying I needed space. Yet, the next morning, when she texted, "I enjoyed our wonderful talk yesterday," followed by photos of her cat, I texted back. To be fair, the cat and I are on good terms. But my mom's message just proved that she didn't catch my "I need space for a while" boundary. I mean, that's probably because I wasn't very good at expressing it *and* totally failed at following through.

Even when you know what boundaries are, what they can do, and why you need them, you can expect two-way malfunctions like this to happen when one person has more power and typically does what they please without consequences, says Dr. Wang.

When you, the one with less say in the dynamic, decide, "Hey, I actually deserve space, respect, and for my preferences to be honored," it "disrupts the dance" the two of you have been doing, explains Dr. Wang.

That's one reason why boundary setting is not a perfect science. Sure, ideally you'd communicate your limit and explain why you're putting it in place, and your mom would welcome it with open arms. But Dr. Wang notes that's not how it works.

For a boundary-setting scenario to play out perfectly, you and your mom would both have to be in an emotionally healthy, regulated place and understand the value of boundaries. If that was your situation, you probably wouldn't be here with me learning how to set boundaries in the first place.

Still, even with those forces working against you, attempting boundary-setting sorcery is worth it. Showing your mom how you want to be treated can protect your individuality, emotions, precious resources, grieving process, and even (potentially) the good parts of your relationship with her.

Here's how to do that, according to Dr. Wang. Results may vary.

Step 1: Get better acquainted with discomfort.

The gateway drug to setting boundaries with your mom is setting boundaries with people who are not your mom.

As we've seen, setting boundaries with momkind can be challenging, especially if you've never tried it, tried and faced backlash, or have been conditioned from birth to please others.

Since setting boundaries is an exercise in vulnerability, practicing with someone you trust and feel safe with is key, says Dr. Wang.

That person could be your partner, a sibling, a close friend, or anyone who loves and understands you, she adds. You could say no to a casual hang you'd normally show up to out of obligation. You could decline doing a favor for your partner. You could call your sister back at a time that's more convenient for you. Those small, low-stakes boundary moments help you tolerate the discomfort of putting yourself first. Over time, that muscle will get stronger.

When in doubt, remind yourself that setting a boundary isn't picking a fight, it's just establishing a system to protect yourself, says Dr. Wang.

Step 2: Brainstorm your boundaries and the consequences.

When you're feeling less intimidated or just sick of dealing with your mom's shenanigans, think about the boundaries you'd like to set. It's helpful to consider which actions really piss you off and the overarching themes that make those behaviors so irritating.

Again, boundaries can be whatever you want them to be. They can range from super flexible (I'll answer the phone when I'm free to talk) to rigid (I will not answer the phone after 8 PM on a weeknight), and they can evolve as needed. For example, maybe it was easy to take your mom's calls when you had a remote gig, but with a new in-office role, you have to change that boundary.

If you're not sure what boundaries make sense in your situation, I have some suggestions later in this chapter (see the *Motherf*cked* Boundary Concierge).

Once you've got a few options, list them from least to most scary. Maybe the easiest one is designating a specific day and time to catch up, and the hardest is not allowing your mom to show up at your house unannounced. Plan to start with the former and work your way to the latter.

You'll also need to enlist enforcers—the things you'll do if your boundaries are crossed. These could be as subtle as not responding to the behavior (ignoring a phone call) or more obvious (leaving in the middle of your lunch date). Try to find an option that's most in line with the problem you're trying to solve. I have some options for how to enforce your boundaries in the Boundary Concierge too.

Step 3: Communicate the boundary.

A quick reminder: You don't have to tell your mom that you're setting a boundary in order to execute it. If that's the best move for you, feel free to skip ahead to Step 6 on page 192.

However, if you plan to stay in contact and want to adjust the way you spend time together, it's helpful if she knows your boundary, says Dr. Wang. Assuming you want to give her a chance—and, again, it's totally fine if you don't—communicating the boundary enables her to make changes that benefit your relationship.

When explaining your boundary, be as clear as possible about where you're drawing the line and what you'll do if it's crossed, says Dr. Wang. Try to get as specific as you can, naming the exact thing you won't put up with and the consequences of doing it.

For example, saying something like "If you say hurtful things about my relationship, I'm going to leave the room" is more tangible and actionable than "You never consider my feelings! Stop being such an asshole, or I'm done!"

If it makes sense for your situation, it can't hurt to use the confrontation sandwich method: Give the positive reason for setting a boundary. Share the boundary and what you'll do if the boundary is crossed. Restate the positive reason for the boundary.

It's also fine to communicate your boundary in a letter or an email, if you're more comfortable with that approach, says Dr. Wang.

You can write something like "Hey Mom, this is something that's been on my mind, and it's very difficult for me to say in person." Then outline your boundary and the consequences. If you're willing to talk about it in person later, make a plan to do so. This is a great option if you're worried your mom's reaction will make you doubt yourself and your boundary when you first share it.

Step 4: Make space for questions and clarifications.

Talking about your limits can be intimidating, and it's possible that you weren't quite as clear as you wanted to be. If you feel safe doing so, consider asking your mom if she has any questions about the boundary and the consequences of stepping over the line.

Allowing her to ask questions gives you the chance to be extra explicit about what you're not tolerating anymore *and* gives your mom a little room to share why abiding by this has been hard for her in the past, says Dr. Wang. That context from your mom may make it easier to give her some grace while she's adjusting to the new rules.

Of course, take whatever she says within the context of your relationship as a whole. If she's been manipulative in the past, it's possible she might use this opportunity to do that now.

Also, this doesn't have to be the last time you ever discuss your boundaries. Go ahead and take some of that pressure off of yourself. Like the rest of the healing process, setting boundaries takes time.

Step 5: If everyone is down for it, create a feedback loop.

You've laid out the boundary and the consequences, made space for questions, and answered them like a damn pro . . . but your mom has proceeded to overstep anyway. This happens, and it doesn't mean the process isn't working.

One way to keep boundary violations from becoming a pattern, though, is to ask your mom if she's open to feedback in real time, says Dr. Wang. That enables her to see how she's being hurtful right away and encourages her to (hopefully) apologize and recalibrate moving forward.

Of course, this feedback loop requires emotional labor on your end, too, and at this point, you might not be willing to put in that work. Still, if your relationship with your mom is mostly good, with just a few areas for improvement—*and* you're down to make the effort—it might help you two interact without the hurtful stuff coming up.

Step 6: Decide when enough is enough.

Sometimes people conflate boundaries with ultimatums, explains Dr. Wang, but these aren't exactly the same. Ultimatums can be much harder on a relationship, and they might not lead to a healthier bond or a better understanding of what's acceptable. An ultimatum is when you say, "Do this thing or I'm completely done with this relationship." Boundaries don't have to be that strict or final.

Long story short, if you want your relationship with your mom to continue, throwing down an ultimatum isn't it. However, if your mom keeps proving that your guardrails mean nothing to her, and the cost of interaction has become too high, it might be time to consider ceasing contact anyway.

To use my crossing-guard analogy again, boundaries allow us to interact with our moms without getting hit by their emotional immaturity. But when Mother plows a minivan through your limits, and that happens over and over, setting boundaries clearly isn't enough to keep you safe. (Apologies for the violence.)

We'll talk more about ending contact in chapter twelve. For now, know that if you feel you need to take drastic measures for your mom to hear you, perhaps the relationship isn't healthy enough to function in the long term.

THE *MOTHERF*CKED* BOUNDARY CONCIERGE

Whether you're out of practice in general or just at a total loss for how to set limits with your mom, creating boundaries can feel much easier in theory than in real life. If you can relate, I bring you the boundary concierge to meet your specific boundary construction needs.

Here, I've provided a list of restrictions to choose from, based on your boundary-setting goal. I also lay out some options for enforcing said boundary, as well as a script you can use to do so. Copy, paste, done!

Instructions

First, skim the Boundaries list, and select one that makes sense for your situation and comfort level. What do you want your boundary to do for you?

Then, choose a Boundary Enforcer that feels most doable—or make up your own.

Last, decide whether you want to communicate this boundary or keep it to yourself. If you'd like to express it to your mom, head down to the Confrontation Sandwich for a script to help you get the boundary from your brain to your mom's. If this boundary is for your mind only, just set that boundary with yourself and go in peace.

Boundaries

The Goal: To gain more independence

Limit the number of times you speak to your mom per week or per month.

Don't answer questions about topics you don't want your mom to know about.

Limit how often you ask your mom for favors or accept money.

Don't discuss new developments in your life (like jobs and relationships) until they reach a specific point of your choosing.

The Goal: To minimize the space your mom takes up in your brain and schedule

Block or mute them on social media.

Limit how much time you spend talking about them with other people.

Limit how much time you spend talking to them on the phone.

Cap how much time you spend with them in person.

Don't let them in your house.

Avoid social events they attend.

The Goal: To avoid the hurtful things your mom says or does

Designate topics, people, or issues you won't talk about.

Make certain parts of your life off limits when you speak.

Cap what topics they can vent to you about.

Choose what you'll let them borrow or take from you.

Decide what activities you won't do with them anymore.

Don't participate in events that felt triggering in the past.

Avoid being alone with them.

The Goal: To protect the good parts of your relationship

Decide what triggering topics you won't discuss.

Decide when and where you are comfortable meeting with them.

Don't allow substance or alcohol use before or during time together.

Make certain parts of your life off limits when you interact.

Ask them to call before coming over.

Boundary Enforcers

Point out the problem and discuss it.

Change the subject.

End the conversation.

Leave the room.

Leave the event.

Cancel existing plans with your mom.

Go home.

Take a timed break.

Ask your mom to leave.

Decline future invitations.

Communicating Your Boundary

You can make boundary setting less unnerving (for everyone involved) by putting it in the middle of a Confrontation Sandwich:

Step 1: Start by explaining the positive reason you're setting this boundary (see: The Goal). Maybe it's for the good of your relationship, but it could also just be beneficial for you.

Step 2: Follow that feel-good moment by describing the boundary you're setting and what you'll do if it's crossed (see: Boundary Enforcers).

Step 3: Reiterate the positive reason you're making this change. Voilà!

Here's the bit to copy and paste:

Hi Mom,

I've been thinking a lot about the parts of our relationship that are working and the ones that leave me feeling [name the emotion]. In order to [state your positive goal], I'd like to start [name your boundary].

If this isn't possible for you, I will [name your Boundary Enforcer]. That said, I'm hoping that this change can [restate positive reason for setting the boundary]. Please let me know if you have any questions. We can talk more about it at [time and place].

CHAPTER 11

Dealing with People Who Don't Get It

When I started to put some distance between my mom and me—calling less frequently, sharing less info about my day-to-day, and so forth—the most stressful part (aside from my mom's reaction) was facing commentary from the family I was closest to. That would be my dad and my nana.

At some point after avoiding my mom on and off for a few months, I called my dad to catch up, as usual. After we chatted for a bit, he asked if I wanted to talk to Foxy. I didn't. But I felt like I couldn't say no.

My dad asked me to do him a solid, so I disappeared my boundaries. I was the good kid! I did what I was told. If I started rebelling now, what would happen to my good standing and perfect attendance? Would my dad think I was a heartless asshole?

I rationalized that I could suck it up for five to ten minutes of my life. So I did. I made small talk and complained to my therapist about it later.

With Nana, my mom's mom and one of my favorite people to ever exist, I tried to avoid any Foxy talk during our regular phone dates, but somehow, my mom's complaints would sneak their way into our conversations anyway. Apparently, Foxy often brought up how I never answer her calls and how I share more with my dad than I do with her.

Your mom isn't the only one who can get in the way of your grieving process and growth. Other people's hot takes on your mom-based loss matter too. They matter so much that there's a whole psychological theory that centers on how feeling misunderstood can impact the grieving process. Disenfranchised grief, anyone?

When the people around you don't see your struggles with your mom as an actual loss, you can feel isolated. You might question whether there's really a problem—especially if those people are your relatives, who have likely known your mom as long as you (if not longer) and have their own ideas about who she is. Their opinions can make you second-guess your emotions. Do they know something you don't? Do their excuses make more sense than your lived experiences? It's disorienting and invalidating.

If you unveil your mom losses to friends or acquaintances, you may find that nobody's reaction is satisfactory. Even if they compare their issues with their mom to yours, you may be left thinking, *Nope, not the same. My mom is much less normal than they think.* Not that you'd tell them and unzip the skin suit covering your true self—the Louis Stevens casing your Malcolm in the Middle innards.

The good news is that you don't *need* social or family support to grow through grief. The bad news is that their support would make that process so much easier. (Some research suggests that our social circles and family culture can accelerate the grieving process, helping us find acceptance and meaning faster.) The neutral news is that you'll be dealing with others' opinions for the foreseeable future.

Those interactions don't have to be detrimental to all the good work you do on your own though. They might even be a fertile testing ground for your grief process. The hypothesis: If you work through your loss in a hotbox of healing, then your growth should hold up in the face of backlash and misunderstanding out in the wild. If you crumble under the pressure to keep up the status quo, maybe you still have some grieving work to do. I'm not a scientist, but that tracks for me.

Family politics are exhausting, but I've learned that the dynamic doesn't change unless you do. Changing requires you believe your feelings, recognize you're grieving something inherently hard to get over (see chapter eight), and use that self-assurance to stand up for yourself. We're healing, we're growing, we're changing. Please clap. When you love yourself more than you love appeasing others, it's so much easier to deal with people who don't get it.

I'm just realizing how simple I made that sound. It's not. Validating your own experiences, traumas, and grief when your bestie doesn't get it, your sister hates that you're bucking the system, and your mom is pissed is a real test. Doing it anyway proves to yourself and anyone who will listen that you deserve to live authentically—even if others don't like what that means for them.

All this gets easier with practice. You realize your family hasn't disowned you for blocking your mom's number. Your best friend doesn't think less of you for feeling bummed throughout Mother's Day season. Or, you realize the worst thing that could happen already did, and you're still here.

In this chapter, I'll explain how to deal with the "other people" part of this process. You'll learn how to handle situations with those who don't get what you're going through (but mean well). And you'll find out how to deal with the people who don't want to see you grow and change.

By the time our work is done here, you'll know how to stick up for yourself and turn these difficult conversations into healing moments. Plus, I've got step-by-step instructions (by now, you know I'm extremely into those) for working through these issues in real time and affirmations for when you're struggling.

DEALING WITH PEOPLE WHO DON'T UNDERSTAND

As we've established, talking about your mom, your big feelings around her, and your healing journey doesn't always feel good. Even if you're venting to someone who wants the best for you, sometimes they just don't relate to your dysfunctional relationship on any level. What a privilege! Good for them, truly. Still, divulging the last unhinged thing your mom did to someone who doesn't get you often makes you feel even worse. More specifically, you might feel judged, misunderstood, insecure, or like a burden.

The thing is, at least in my experience, your closest friends, chosen family, or whoever you're confiding in probably isn't judging or feeling burdened by you. That call is likely coming from inside the house. In reality, your people probably feel for you and want to see you happy but just can't understand your situation.

That makes sense though, right? You are the only one who has fully experienced this relationship with your mom. How *could* they get it to the full extent you'd like them to? I used to tell my therapist that I wished I had a clone of myself who experienced my mom in the exact way I did. Then I'd have someone to confirm my suspicions that a lot of this stuff was, in fact, fucked up.

All that said, this dynamic can also happen between you and people who are more familiar with your mom drama (or your mom in general). Whether it's your sibling, cousin, or grandparent, some people can't acknowledge what you're going through because it would disrupt the way they live, says Whitney Goodman, creator of the Calling Home community and podcast.

"Someone could be in denial for their own protective reasons. That's especially true for a sibling, because seeing it from your perspective would complicate their life or make them feel something negative," she explains. Preach.

Here's what to do with people who resist seeing your side or just don't get it.

Step 1: Assess your capacity for unhelpful feedback and triggering interactions.

The easiest way to navigate conversations with people who don't understand what you're going through is to keep triggering conversations off the table. If you're in the early days of your grieving/healing journey, this move could be especially helpful, says Goodman.

That's because, as you know, you're more likely to question your feelings and perspective when you first start addressing a painful relationship with your mom. So the chances of you accidentally gaslighting yourself are much higher, she adds.

Check in with yourself. You can journal or just sit with questions like, *How will I feel if their response isn't exactly what I need it to be? Is it even possible for them to react the right way, or are my expectations too high? Am I still questioning whether my feelings about my mom are justified? Could their response to me venting or sharing information about my relationship with my mom make me second-guess myself?*

If the answer to any of these questions is yes, proceed with caution. Also, again, if you're not already seeing a therapist, do that! They're a great unbiased resource. You shouldn't be going through this on your own.

Step 2: Censor yourself.

Even if you're just getting started in the grieving process, you don't have to take a vow of silence. But it may be useful to limit what you share with other people, if you're worried about their response. This is especially helpful when you're kind of on the fence about whether talking about your mom will make you un-believe yourself.

You can also experiment, gathering more emotional data to figure out who to avoid talking about your mom with. Worried about how your best friend will respond? Text them some of the crazy things your maternal figure does in real time and see how they react. If they're shocked, you might feel validated. If they try to make excuses for your mom, though, maybe they're not the right outlet. Data point established.

Say you're rehashing childhood memories with your sister, and they laugh off how your mom used to "beat your asses" when you were mischievous. You could respond with "You know, that was really hurtful, and I'm still having a hard time recovering from it." If they still act like it wasn't a big deal, then there you have it—declare that space unsafe.

However, if your sister seems open to your perspective, you can dip your toe into that convo to get a sense of where their head is. You'll also want to pay attention to how you feel when that chat is over. Are you more confused than when you started? If so, then that's another sign this topic should be off limits with your sis for now.

Step 3: Be your own source of support.

You shouldn't go it alone on this motherfucked journey. Therapy, close friends, chosen family, and virtual group support are all great reinforcements. Yet, to grow, you have to establish a sense of security within yourself. Then you can face people who don't understand, tell your truth, and not feel weird about it.

It would be impossible to avoid closeness with anyone who doesn't appreciate what it's like to have a dysfunctional relationship with your mom. Remind yourself that it's all right if people don't realize what you're going through. It's OK if they're not sure how to support you the way you'd like. You don't need their validation to believe yourself. It's real because it happened to you. You know what's true for you, says Goodman.

Reassuring yourself like this is a vital part of healing from your relationship with your mom, she adds. When compounded with all the assignments from chapter eight, you'll be on your way to feeling better.

DEALING WITH PEOPLE WHO HATE GROWTH

There's a big difference between those who don't know what you're dealing with and those who actively discourage you from working through it.

The latter are people I like to think of as Growth Haters. As 3LW taught us, haters are going to hate. I'm sure the Growth Haters in your life are mostly good people. But when confronted with your mom-based grief, emotions, and experiences, they say, "Nope. Not today." They might even try to convince you you're wrong.

Oftentimes, these people come in the form of family or even family friends. If your family culture emphasizes the importance of tradition and your role within this group, breaking patterns can feel intimidating. That's true for you and the fine people you call family. When we're so used to functioning in a specific way that upholds family dysfunction, it's hard to stop. We might not even notice we're enabling bad behavior.

That's disorienting as hell and gets in the way of the massive internal work you've been doing on your own. Here's how to deal when confronted by this group of people, family or not.

Step 1: Reflect on your sense of safety.

You're not starting from scratch here. You probably have a sense of how your family responds to people who go against the grain. Maybe you've heard them talking shit about your "self-centered" cousins or "too-good-for-us" uncle. That family gossip will get to you, for sure. It also exposes the danger zones for discussing your mom drama.

You should also think about how they respond to your mom's chaos. Do they appease them? Do they make excuses for them? Do they just try to ignore it? Or perhaps they show signs that they've had it with your mom as well. Have they set boundaries or found ways to navigate the situation? These are data points, too, my friends.

Last, think about the times you've spoken about your mom with this person or the hurtful interactions they've been around to witness. How did they respond? More importantly, how did their response leave you feeling?

Step 2: Test the waters.

If that little thought exercise made you realize this person isn't a safe place for your mom complaints, skip ahead to Step 3. See you soon.

Sometimes, it's hard to tell how the fam will respond to your expression of mother displeasure. If you're getting mixed signals, it can't hurt to do a little experimenting here.

Ditto if there are family members you interact with frequently or can't avoid. Even if you suspect they won't be receptive, giving them a shot can shed light on how to navigate those relationships in a strategic way. The more you know, you know?

When you're in a place that feels emotionally and physically safe, bring up your mom. You can mention a recent thing they did that hurt your feelings, a statement about your relationship in general, or some option I'm not thinking of. But resist the urge to unload or go off just yet. This is a test.

As in the previous step, your assignment is to think about how interacting with that person left you feeling. If you started to doubt yourself or felt compelled to argue your case, you could probably use some boundaries (see Step 3).

On the flip side, if they seemed open and interested in your perspective, that's a good sign! Just proceed with caution and make sure you're confiding in someone you really trust and who has your back. You can always decide to censor yourself or set boundaries later if it starts to feel uncomfortable.

Step 3: Establish boundaries.

When your family or family friends or whoever is hating on your growth trajectory, setting limits can help you stay close (or close enough) while guarding your grief.

But first, let's cultivate some empathy. This person is doing what they feel is most protective for them, just like you are, says Goodman. There's nothing wrong with that, even if you don't agree. Perhaps this perspective makes their opposition feel less personal, which is always helpful.

Next, think about how you can safely interact with them. What could your relationship look like if you deleted your mom from the equation? Maybe you could have some quality one-on-one time where Mother doesn't come up.

However, if they can't separate you from your situation with your mom, that's a sign you need to take more serious measures. For example, if they won't stop bringing her up, trying to act as your mom's personal representative, or reporting everything you say back to her, it's time to verbalize your boundaries.

Technically speaking, censoring yourself is setting a boundary. Remember, you don't need to Declare a Boundary for it to exist. However, if the other person doesn't catch on to your mom omissions, you'll need to use your words.

Here's how, according to Goodman: Say something like "I know you're trying to help, but for us to have a good relationship, we can't talk about my mom or the issues I'm having with her. Do you think we can do that? I need to deal with this on my own right now."

Hopefully, they take it in stride, give it their best shot, and apologize if they genuinely forget the new rules of engagement. Try to have patience here.

Step 4: Take some space (at least for now).

Of course, sometimes your relatives or family friends won't comply at all. When that happens, it's totally fine to pull back for a bit, says Goodman. This is especially true in those early days, when you're still low-key doubting whether your feelings and experiences are real.

Once you feel like you can believe yourself and your grief, it's easier to reconcile that other people have different experiences. "I think that's the biggest challenge that we have to face in families with dysfunction," Goodman explains. "We're all going to have different experiences of that dysfunction."

Though it's hard to hold your truth and others' at once, doing so is a major sign of progress. It also makes engaging with different perspectives more manageable.

AFFIRMATIONS FOR TRUSTING YOURSELF

Believing the reality of your relationship with your mom and the way it makes you feel is hard. That's especially true if your mom or other people consistently downplay your feelings.

Accepting who your mom is and your relationship with them requires trusting your gut. You can't do all that good grief work without first admitting you lost something. To help you help yourself, here are a few realistic yet positive affirmations to establish some confidence when other people's opinions are louder than your own experience. Use them before a difficult conversation or to feel more supported afterward. Enjoy!

I know what's true, even if no one else does.

Everyone has their own experience of my mom and my relationship with her, and that doesn't change my reality.

My truth and other people's will never be the same, but there's room for all of them.

It's perfectly OK if I'm the only one who believes me.

Not everyone will understand what I'm going through, but I still do.

Only I get to decide how much I owe my mom.

The more I believe in myself, the closer I get to acceptance.

My feelings about my mom are real, and nobody's opinion changes that.

I can give myself all the validation I need to move through this challenging time.

Make your own: Even though ____ [obstacle you're facing], I ____ [your ideal outcome] ____.

CHAPTER 12
How to Do Estrangement

Up until the last few years, estrangement (also called going low- or no-contact) wasn't a thing I heard much about. These days, though, as a mental health editor and writer and a person on the internet, I've noticed a massive uptick in search traffic and social media interest around the subject—and in the number of people willing to talk about it.

Another thing that happened in the last few years: I became estranged from my mom.

It wasn't something I ever considered previously. I told myself that the things my mom did or said didn't warrant it. I thought estrangement was for people who were treated far worse than I was. As a kid, I was fed, clothed, and taken to school. My mom drove me to dance class and let me host sleepovers. I'm pretty sure I've never even been spanked.

I now know that mistreatment doesn't have to be illegal to be abuse (see chapter four). I also know that my mom didn't meet my emotional needs. I was parentified and taught that my feelings don't matter. Those lessons went on to impact the way I showed up at work and in my friendships. They also convinced me that putting my feelings aside so my mom could have her ideal mother–child relationship was the way it had to be.

On top of all that, the idea of becoming someone who's estranged from their mom made me feel physically dirty. Stigma is weird, man.

I spent five years in therapy circling the drain of hurtful interactions with my mom. I made excuses for her, like "This is just her personality!" and "She means well!"

I made excuses for myself too. *Protecting my feelings isn't worth it. She's not going to change, so boundaries are pointless.* I avoided the root of the problem and confrontation. I refused to break out of my eldest-daughter role (if you know, you know). I refused to believe myself.

The moment I knew I had to change how this dynamic was dynamicing came months after I told my mom how I felt about our relationship (for those playing along at home, this would be my State of the Relationship Speech). At that point, I had been blocking my mom's number on and off for months, yet I was still consumed by our relationship. I thought about her more often than not. I could hear her passive-aggressive comments in my head. I cautiously navigated my relationships with the people we had in common. I vented endlessly to Sean and any friend who'd hear me out—all while seeing a therapist every other week. This shit was so monotonous. I was sick of myself.

Finally, I figured out that every time my mom reached out to me, it made it harder to move on.

Now that I know more about grief, this makes so much sense, right? Whenever Foxy called me and left a chirpy voicemail that shamed me for not answering (a strange combination, honestly), I doubted myself. Was I making this a bigger deal than it was? Her tone of voice sounded so excited, so why did I feel so awful?

Turns out, the cognitive dissonance between the state of our relationship (bad) and how she sounded on the phone (alarmingly positive) hurt my brain and my feelings. I couldn't get out of grief mode and back into life mode when the person causing the grief called every week. Ambiguous loss is such an asshole.

Once I realized staying in contact was keeping me stuck, I decided I had to change. This epiphany is my free gift with purchase to you.

In this chapter, we'll break down the nuances of estrangement, including what it really means, who it's for, who it's not, and how to decide what's best for you. I also talked to Whitney Goodman—someone who sees estrangement all the time in her practice and therapy groups—about the best way to go about this process.

Whether you're already considering this arrangement or not, I'd like to kindly suggest you stick around to learn more about estrangement, if only for your friends who might be going through it. Your understanding and support can make this painful decision more bearable for anyone forced to choose it.

WHAT IS ESTRANGEMENT?

The APA describes estrangement as "a significant decrease or discontinuation of contact with individuals with whom one formerly had close relationships, such as a spouse or family member, due to apathy or antagonism."

So that's the official definition we're working with, but you'll notice it's still a little vague. How much is a "significant" decrease? What do they mean by "close"? And does estrangement only happen because we're not interested in this person anymore or we're actively fighting? Respectfully, I don't think so.

Goodman says everyone engaged in estrangement will have a different definition of what it means and looks like for them. In general, though, she says estrangement is a temporary or permanent ending of a relationship for a reason. Usually, it's with family. This setup is also sometimes called going low-contact or no-contact.

For some, low-contact means staying in touch but with minimal contact. You might check in via text, email, quarterly phone calls, or greeting cards. Or you could catch up more frequently but avoid sharing the details of your life (you might be doing this already). Some would say talking once a week with the person is low-contact to them, says Goodman; others might say once a year.

No-contact also isn't as clear as it sounds. You could have your mom's phone number blocked but allow them to reach you via email or social media. Or you could block them on everything and stay cordial at big family events. Alternately, your version of no-contact could be straight up avoiding them on every level. There really aren't any rules on what this looks like. It's up to you.

If this sounds a lot like our discussion on boundaries, you're right! I've come to understand going low- or no-contact as just unlocking the next level of boundary work—a framing that feels less scary and is probably even healthy.

A quick refresher on boundaries: They permit us to separate what we're willing to put up with from what we're not. They're meant to protect who we are, how we feel, our energy, and our resources. When it comes to your relationship with your mom, your boundaries can be as understated as not replying to certain emails or as big as blocking all communication.

Boundaries allow us to engage in relationships in a way that keeps us safe. However, if your maternal figure keeps blowing through the rules you set, estrangement becomes a useful option. Think of it as a high-intensity kind of boundary you establish to protect yourself, especially when other boundaries fail. It might not be a fit for everyone, but it can be a game-changer for those who've unsuccessfully tried to navigate their relationship with their caregiver.

As with any boundary, estrangement isn't meant to teach your caregiver a lesson. It's meant to keep you safe so you can grieve, heal, and accept your relationship with your mom for what it is.

Lots of parents of estranged adult kids subscribe to a narrative in which estrangement is just a trendy way for young people to punish their parents impulsively after being brainwashed by their therapists or social media. But I couldn't find any research that supports this view, and Goodman says she's never met a single person who used estrangement in this way.

WHO IS ESTRANGEMENT FOR?

First, let's discuss who it's not for. Goodman says that if going low- to no-contact with your mom will inhibit your connection to other healthy family relationships, important gatherings, money, community, or your culture, perhaps this isn't the right move. You don't want to lose all your sources of support as you navigate a dysfunctional relationship with your mom. Sometimes, it's not worth managing one part of your life by blowing up the others.

That said, don't abandon your other boundaries! Those will keep you safe and sane as you process this relationship. Then, you can find other, more helpful modes of protection. You might take space from your mom in less restrictive ways or try to make peace with a more surface-level dynamic. Continue experimenting until you find what works.

However, if going low- or no-contact will not have a deleterious effect on your well-being and might, in fact, enhance it, this option might be for you.

When moms refuse to take accountability, apologize, or show that they're willing to stop hurting you, ceasing and desisting contact provides a protective shield. And for people who've been emotionally, physically, mentally, financially, or even spiritually abused by their moms, this could be the best option to avoid future mistreatment.

Even if you wouldn't categorize your mom's treatment as abuse, escalating to a low- or no-contact situation could still be the next logical step, says Goodman. You've set limitations, tried to find common ground, confronted your mom about how her behavior impacts you, and waited for her to use your feedback. If she keeps on keeping on, you might decide to end communication with her.

Say you aren't OK with a superficial maternal relationship, but your mom refuses to delve deeper. Going low- or no-contact is also an option for you. As with any other relationship, you can opt out of what doesn't make you feel good. It's fine to want a stronger emotional connection with your mom. And it's more than fine to walk away when you don't get it. You decide what kinds of relationships you foster and which you don't. The title of "mom" doesn't change that.

What I'm saying is that "tried everything" also means "tried everything you're willing to try." There's no criteria you need to fulfill to qualify for estrangement. Being tired of the monotony is enough.

A VERY UNOFFICIAL ESTRANGEMENT READINESS ASSESSMENT

Though these questions are based on my interviews with Whitney Goodman, a licensed therapist, I am not a mental health pro—and this is not a diagnostic tool. So please take this quiz with a large grain of salt. Still, if you're wondering whether going low- or no-contact could help you solve your mom situation, answering these questions could bring some clarity.

Instructions

For each of the statements below, circle the number that aligns with your perspective right now. When you're done, add up the numbers and divide them by 20. You can come back to this quiz anytime as you think through whether estrangement is right for you.

1. **I've tried to set boundaries, but my mom doesn't abide by them.**

   strongly disagree 1 2 3 4 5 strongly agree

2. **There are many things I don't share with my mom.**

   strongly disagree 1 2 3 4 5 strongly agree

3. **Mentally preparing to spend time with my mom takes so much energy.**

   strongly disagree 1 2 3 4 5 strongly agree

4. **Ending contact with my mom would mean ending relationships with other family members with whom I have a healthy relationship.**

   strongly agree 1 2 3 4 5 strongly disagree

5. **I have a hard time enforcing my boundaries because my mom keeps overstepping.**

   strongly disagree 1 2 3 4 5 strongly agree

6. **After spending time with my mom, I feel mentally and/or emotionally exhausted.**

   strongly disagree 1 2 3 4 5 strongly agree

7. **I've cut back on the time I spend with my mom, but I don't feel any better.**

   strongly disagree 1 2 3 4 5 strongly agree

8. **It's hard for me to name the things I gain from my relationship with my mom.**

   strongly disagree 1 2 3 4 5 strongly agree

9. **I'll lose access to financial support that I need if I go low- or no-contact with my mom.**

   strongly agree 1 2 3 4 5 strongly disagree

10. **Managing conflict with my mom (or the repercussions of it) impacts how much time I have for myself, my partner, my kids, and/or my work.**

    strongly disagree 1 2 3 4 5 strongly agree

11. **I spend too much time arguing with my mom in my head.**

    strongly disagree 1 2 3 4 5 strongly agree

12. **I'm sick of always venting about my mom.**

    strongly disagree 1 2 3 4 5 strongly agree

13. **Guilt and obligation hold me back from spending less energy on my mom.**

    strongly disagree 1 2 3 4 5 strongly agree

14. **I've blocked my mom on some platforms, but she always finds ways to reach me.**

    strongly disagree 1 2 3 4 5 strongly agree

15. **Even though I've expressed my feelings, my mom rarely or never takes accountability for the ways she's hurt me.**

    strongly disagree 1 2 3 4 5 strongly agree

16. **When I took a break from being in contact with my mom in the past, I felt less preoccupied by our relationship.**

    strongly disagree 1 2 3 4 5 strongly agree

17. **I hope that cutting off my mom will encourage her to become the person I wish she was.**

    strongly agree 1 2 3 4 5 strongly disagree

18. **My mom complains about my existing boundaries to me and others who tell me about it.**

    strongly disagree 1 2 3 4 5 strongly agree

19. **My mom finds ways to use my boundaries against me.**

    strongly disagree 1 2 3 4 5 strongly agree

20. **If I'm estranged from my mom, I'll miss out on important parts of my culture or community.**

    strongly agree 1 2 3 4 5 strongly disagree

TOTAL SCORE ____ DIVIDED BY 20 = ____

Results

If you scored less a 3 or less: There may actually be plenty of reasons to stay in touch with your mom. When she's your connection to resources or community, losing those things might take a bigger toll on your well-being than enduring some contact with your mom to maintain this connection. Family, money, and your culture might even support you as you grieve the things your mom will never be, says Goodman.

Try taking an inventory of the limits you already set with your mom. It's possible she needs clear communication about the kind of interactions you will and will not tolerate. Give it a try! Her response will tell you more about the next steps you need to take. The more she tolerates your limits, the less likely you'll need estrangement in order to start feeling better.

If you scored higher than 3: Estrangement might make sense in your situation. What it ultimately comes down to is weighing what you have to lose against what you gain by staying in this relationship. That can take years of experimenting to figure out.

Here's the general guideline, though: If you've put limits in place, restricted the things you talk about, and limited how much you see each other, but your mom crashes through those boundaries like they don't exist, further limiting her access to you can bring some peace, says Goodman. This isn't an easy decision, so spend time with your journal, an objective friend, or a mental health professional (maybe all three) to sort it out.

Whether you decide estrangement is the right move for you or not, keep reading to determine the best way to go about it.

HOW TO GO LOW- OR NO-CONTACT

Methods of pursuing estrangement aren't restricted to blocking numbers, emails, and socials. Goodman says that, ideally, this process is a series of experiments where you try new strategies to see what feels good and what doesn't. Then you can use that info to move forward. It's about discovering what works for you.

Here are some steps that can help you do that.

Step 1: Decide how much contact you want.

Sure, terms like "low-contact" and "no-contact" might imply that you need to drop yourself into a cute little category and stay there, but don't get hung up on labels. The most important part is deciding how you want to communicate and how often, says Goodman.

To start this process, think about how much contact you have now. How often do you spend time together? What does that time look like? What would you change to make this relationship less taxing?

Maybe you see your mom every Sunday, let them come over whenever, and answer all of their texts—even the ones you don't want to. Consider which of these interactions takes the most out of you, and ask yourself, *Would eliminating that point of contact make the relationship less exhausting overall?*

As with chapter nine's boundary-setting steps, you can begin to reclaim some space by tackling the easiest restrictions first. For example, in the scenario I just described, you might decide that you're going to check in with yourself before determining if and when you'll text back.

If that tweak to your dynamic makes you feel content, that's a success, and you can stop there. If not, it could be worth taking additional steps.

For those who've been laying down boundaries for a while now, such steps could look like taking a quick inventory of the limits you've already set up and how those are working (or aren't). Honestly, if you're considering estrangement, that inventory is probably quite the list.

Say you're screening their phone calls, being selective about sharing life details, and only spending time together in a group setting. Is your mom able to abide by those rules? Is she attempting to make you feel guilty for setting them?

By considering what works best for you and whether your mom will play by those rules, you can develop a plan that fosters maximum chill without fully leaving the relationship, Goodman says.

This boundary adjustment process may be long and slow, but armed with additional data points, you can make well-informed decisions you feel good about.

Step 2: Communicate your decision (or not).

Explaining your boundaries requires you to stand up for yourself and trust that you're doing the best thing for you and this relationship (or lack thereof).

But, again, you don't have to formally announce you're going low- or no-contact. In some situations, laying out your plans and why you put them in place can be pointless at best and harmful at worst.

When your version of low- or no-contact doesn't require that your mom start or stop doing something, you don't need to tell them you're doing it, says Goodman. You can hold back information about your life or avoid certain events without talking about it. Your mom might notice and ask what's going on, and if she does, you can tell her why you're not getting into your dating life or attending the family reunion. But you don't have to. You're welcome to make excuses or just say, "Yep, you're right, I'm not doing that anymore." You don't owe her an explanation.

The same is true if your mom has distanced herself already. Maybe she's not calling to check in, attempting to spend time with you, or otherwise making any effort to stay in touch. In that case, reaching out to say, "Hey, just so you know, I need a break," isn't helpful.

Often, Goodman says, people reach out to request space from someone who's distanced themselves because they're looking for the other person to come back and say, "Hey, wait! I love you and want to work on this relationship!" While that hope is so real, threatening to go no-contact for that reason might leave you more hurt and disappointed than you already are.

When the relationship is volatile or abusive, telling your mom that you're cutting back on contact can be dangerous, says Goodman. "We wouldn't recommend doing that in domestic violence situations or any other type of abusive relationship," she explains. "I don't think that changes when it's between you and your parent. You should always prioritize safety in your unique situation." Mental and emotional safety count, too, by the way.

So when *do* you need to inform your mom of your decision to take space? If you're not worried about your safety, your mom hasn't left the chat, and your boundaries require your mom to change her behavior, then go for it. That might look like asking her to stop coming over without calling first or telling her that you don't want any gifts this holiday season.

Sharing your decision with your mom also makes sense if your boundary drastically changes the way you two interact, like if you and your mom usually talk every day but you've decided to stop speaking to them altogether, says Goodman.

Here's how to go about communicating your low- or no-contact status: While you can absolutely use the State of the Relationship Speech or Classic Q&A methods from chapter nine here, you don't have to get that intense.

You've probably explained to your mom the ways she's hurt you many, many times before, says Goodman. Even if you haven't explicitly pointed out every single occasion she hurt your feelings, your body language and tone of voice likely have conveyed how her actions impacted you. If you're tired of retelling those painful events, consider this your permission not to.

Whether you decide to get into the minutiae of your issues with your mom or not, think about the communication modality that makes you feel safest. It could be a letter, phone call, or in person. Whatever feels most accessible to you is fair game, says Goodman.

Next, plan what you want to say. This can, and probably should, be worded in an easy-to-understand, pragmatic, factual way, says Goodman. If you're unsure how to go about that, just draft up what you're going to do (not speak on the phone, visit less often, etc.), why you're doing it (I'm tired of being bullied, you don't respect my choices), and what you need from them (don't leave voicemails, don't come over unannounced, try to respect my decision).

Yeah, this may seem relatively straightforward, but don't be surprised if you have a difficult time. Distilling a lifetime of issues into a few sentences is tough.

Then, it's time to mentally prepare for your delivery. You want to be calm, professional, and emotionally mature. Doing so will equalize the power dynamic. Think of it as showing up as a representative of yourself rather than coming in hot with your heart on your sleeve and making yourself more vulnerable.

This approach also minimizes your mom's ability to use anything you say against you. "I know it's awful to say to a victim, 'You need to show up professionally in front of your abuser,'" says Goodman. "But the reality is they have the power to utilize those feelings against you." Showing up as your professional self is a form of self-protection.

Before you tell your mom what's up, spend some time venting your anger and frustrations to someone you trust or your journal to keep your emotions from getting the best of you. Your feelings matter. But after sharing them with your mom time and time again, to no effect, you know emotions won't be helpful here.

Once you're ready (or ready enough) to tell your mom how you'll be communicating with her going forward, do it.

Step 3: Keep track of how you feel.

You've decided what low- or no-contact looks like for you, and you've expressed that in the most emotionally mature way possible (or decided against saying anything at all). So now you're done here, yes?

Well, not exactly. What comes next is the whole point of this experiment: noticing what your life feels like with less of your mom in it. Goodman says the best way to tell how estrangement is working for you is to check in with how you're feeling as much as you can. Keep a journal, track your feelings in an app (like Dr. Marc Brackett's How We Feel app), take voice notes . . . you get the idea. Just spend time with your feelings and keep an eye on how they change.

Yes, the feelings you're tracking can be related to your mom and how much contact you have with her, but don't forget about all the others, says Goodman. That's because it might not be obvious which feelings are related to your maternal figure and which aren't. For example, after breaking patterns that existed for a long time, you might get a sense that something is off. Maybe you feel purposeless or lost. Maybe it's like you left something at home on your way to the airport, but don't know what it is.

All of that is normal, says Goodman. So is feeling like you really miss your mom, even if you know you did the right thing. Of course, everyone's situation is different. Maybe you don't truly miss *her*, but miss the idea of a person she'll never be. By losing touch with your mom, you're also extinguishing the fantasy that things will get better in the right circumstances.

If this estrangement thing is working, though, those feelings should start to come up less frequently and/or become less intense, she adds. At the same time, you'll likely feel some relief. You could notice more peace in your life and more space to focus on other things. You could have more energy for relationships that used to take a backseat or were dominated by venting about your mom.

Most importantly, you'll have space to grieve what you lost in your dysfunctional relationship with your mom, and who your mom will never be, while getting closer to acceptance. It's painful work, but it can be easier when you're not reminded of your loss all the damn time.

When I blocked my mom's number for the last time, I didn't feel that great at first. I tried to remember that she wasn't willing to meet me where I needed her. She wanted the perks of a close relationship, like regular phone calls, walking me down the aisle, and headlines about my life she could share with her friends. She wanted to visit me so she could see "the sights" and post about it on Facebook. She was happy with a surface-level relationship, but maintaining it meant sacrificing my needs. I wasn't willing to go along with her version of a "good" relationship anymore.

When she couldn't reach me, I didn't have to worry if she'd call me or leave voicemails. I didn't hang up the phone and burst into tears. I didn't spend as much time venting about Foxy to anyone who'd listen. I didn't have to pretend this relationship was normal and fine.

That said, estrangement can't fix everything. Even if you're taking the most space possible from your mom, the damage that relationship has done remains, says Goodman. The emotional and mental impact won't go away just because she isn't blowing up your phone. "Certainly, with distance, you're going to feel some improvement," she explains. "But if we're talking about things that have been going on since childhood, I don't think estrangement is enough to fix that."

In cases of abuse or serious mistreatment, you could have developed conditions like anxiety, depression, posttraumatic stress disorder, or complex posttraumatic stress disorder, says Goodman. Plus, as we know from part one, the way our moms treat us can affect how we see ourselves, the world, and our place in it—with or without a mental health diagnosis.

Estrangement probably won't make you stop wanting your mom either. Whether you've been estranged for two months, two years, or two decades, wanting a maternal presence to be there for you, have your back, and love you unconditionally likely won't go away, says Goodman.

That's why the grieving process is so useful. Working through those losses, perhaps with the help of a professional, can help you find some contentment even if the cravings never fully evaporate.

YET ANOTHER REMINDER: A THERAPIST CAN HELP!

If, during estrangement, you notice that you're having more bad days than good, your mom stuff is starting to interfere with your other relationships, your job, or any other important part of your life, it's time to seek out a mental health pro who can help you navigate all that.

If you're open to it, having a therapist early on in this process, like before you even start pulling back from your relationship with your mom, can make this whole thing easier. You'll have an objective person who can help you sort through the complicated feelings about your mom, this relationship, and what you want to do with it. They can assist every step of the way.

Step 4: Get through the guilt.

In his book, *Permission to Feel,* psychologist Dr. Marc Brackett explains that guilt happens when we judge ourselves for doing something that feels wrong. We feel responsible for that bad thing and are remorseful that it happened.

Most of the time, we feel guilt when we act in ways that go against our moral character or our values. Guilt lets us know that we might need to make things right with someone we hurt and avoid doing that again.

When you're entering the low- to no-contact era of your relationship with your mom, you will probably feel some guilt. But that doesn't mean you've done anything wrong.

Oftentimes, this guilt stems from being conditioned to take care of your mom's feelings, says Goodman. You might even believe you're abandoning her if you don't continue doing it. The fact that the relationship is unhealthy and harmful doesn't always matter.

If you're feeling intense guilt, that might indicate that you could use some help working through your emotions so you don't make any rash decisions. "In those moments, it's really good to have a therapist or a group or somebody to help you understand where that feeling is coming from," says Goodman. They can remind you that you're doing what's best for you, and you're not responsible for your mom's feelings.

For now, remember that you probably wouldn't stick with a friend or a partner who treated you this shitty, so why make an exception for your mom? Try thinking about that the next time the guilt hits.

Step 5: Adjust your boundaries as needed.

As with any boundary, you can always tweak how much contact you have with your mom.

Ideally, this involves a continuous assessment of what works and what doesn't. But in a lot of cases, Goodman says, the best method for going low- or no-contact is choosing the least intense version you can manage, communicating it, giving it time to evolve, and figuring out how you feel after it's in place. In other words, use the same steps that brought you to choose estrangement in the first place.

If the low-contact plan you've established feels sustainable and makes you less obsessive or overwhelmed by the relationship, *and* your mom is able to abide by your rules, you might have found a solution. Success!

If it doesn't keep your mom from belittling you, violating your boundaries, emotionally manipulating you, or abusing you, you could level up. The same goes if your remaining interactions leave you feeling drained, anxious, or depressed, says Goodman.

"If low-contact is not successful, you can of course pull back further," she explains. "There are a lot of people in this situation who realize going low-contact isn't working because the other person continues to demand more."

There's also the possibility that you went low-contact and your mom responded by going no-contact, says Goodman. In that case, the estrangement is happening to you, she adds. If you can relate, take a beat to see how you feel. Even if the decision wasn't yours, the space could make you feel more at ease. Perhaps they did the hard part for you?

After being low- or no-contact for a while, you might start feeling so good that you wonder if it's worth getting back in touch with your mom. The same could also happen if you just really miss having a mom in your life.

If you consider resuming contact, Goodman says to ask yourself, *What's changed?* Has your mom started going to therapy, working on herself, and apologizing to other family members she hurt? Did she write you a letter explaining how she knows she messed up your relationship and she's willing to work to make amends? Most importantly, is there any indisputable evidence that things will be different if you let her back into your life?

If the answer is no, you can also ask yourself, *Have I changed*? Have you healed to the point that you can better manage interactions with her, prioritize your needs, and protect yourself against any hurtful behavior? That's possible too. Maybe after a few years, her manipulation won't affect you the same. You'll think, *What a weird thing to say out loud*, and move on with your day. If so, maybe estrangement is no longer necessary.

"I always like to tell people that if and when the facts change, you can do something different. Until that happens, staying estranged might be the best decision for some people," says Goodman.

GREEN FLAGS FOR GETTING BACK IN TOUCH

Thinking about reaching out to your mom after going low- or no-contact and looking for more explicit direction? Nice! Ultimately, the choice to reengage your mom is yours, and you can reach out for any reason that seems important enough to you.

That said, these are the biggest indicators that your relationship could look and feel different once you reconnect, according to Goodman.

- Your mom is actively doing the work, and others say she's making strides.
- Your mom apologizes genuinely for the ways she's hurt you, naming what she did and how she affected you.
- Your mom stopped the harmful behavior you asked her to quit (substance misuse, gambling, yelling, etc.).

- Your mom admits fault and no longer blames external factors for her behavior.
- You feel less triggered by your mom's behavior.
- The benefits of spending time with your mom now outweigh the risks.
- You have a new infrastructure in place to support you when your mom inevitably acts out.
- You're willing to have a surface-level relationship with your mom.
- You are prepared to stand up for yourself and defend against unhealthy, harmful, or manipulative behavior.

SOME MOMS WILL NEVER UNDERSTAND WHY YOU'RE ESTRANGED

After I went no-contact, my mom started to take up less mental space. Over time, there was more room up there for me to be with my feelings without interference. My own voice finally got louder than the sound of hers.

Today, I barely clock her chaos. Last Christmas, my mom gave me regifted candy from her volunteer job (the tag read "From: ~~hospice~~ mom"). Also included: previously worn Santa socks and a well-used eyebrow pencil. I told her not to get me anything a long time ago, but I suppose she was in the holiday spirit.

Instead of feeling shitty, misunderstood, and disappointed, I laughed and added it to a file in my brain named "Evidence that this relationship is weird."

That said, this is not a paid endorsement of estrangement. It makes me sad that not talking to my mom feels better. I sincerely wish this wasn't the solution to being otherwise consumed by feelings about Foxy, but for now it is.

As you might have guessed, my mom doesn't seem to understand why I put our low-contact arrangement in place. And your mom might not either. You can tell her how she hurt you, set boundaries, explain why you're putting them in place, go low- or no-contact, and explain why you're doing that, but your mom may never comprehend what they're doing wrong.

When I finally went low- to no-contact, it was after years of slowly pulling away. I'd told my mom over and over how she'd hurt my feelings, that I felt like she didn't want to spend time with or get to know me. When my family relayed that Foxy didn't know what the problem was, I went ahead and emailed the list of bullet points I'd read to her over the phone months earlier. If she still doesn't get it, that's fine with me.

It's not just Foxy out here staying confused. Some studies suggest it's relatively common for estranged parents to have a completely different perspective on why their adult kid left the relationship. Maybe you won't be surprised to learn that the parents surveyed were unlikely to reflect on the part they played in estrangement.

For example, in one survey of more than a thousand moms who were estranged from their adult children, researchers found that these moms tended to report that external factors were to blame for the state of their relationship. Those reasons included kids being turned against them by other family members or romantic partners, and the adult child's mental health.

In general, moms in this study were less likely to blame "internal attributions for estrangement" compared to "external attributions." They were also less likely to "validate their children's complaints about abuse or neglect."

Another survey examining parents' and adult children's reasons for estrangement had similar results. Moms and dads blamed the distance on their kids' relationships with others and "sense of entitlement." The parents surveyed were also more likely to say they weren't sure why their kids were estranged from them.

Listen, I'm not here to say these people are narcissistic monsters who hate emotional maturity and joy. The experts I spoke with all agree that it's hard for moms (or parents in general) to shift their behavior or see the hurt they've caused after years of perpetrating it. It takes a lot of courage and humility to do that.

My point is to remind you that your mom doesn't have to understand why you're estranging yourself for this process to be healing. The only person who needs to fully get it is you.

CHAPTER 13

*What Motherf*cking Growth Feels Like*

If this book does anything for you, I hope it makes you feel seen, supported, and part of a community you didn't know existed. You're not the only one who hasn't always (or ever) felt great about your mom. You're not the only one who is held back by motherfucked relationships or trauma. You're also not the only one trying to heal—and probably pissing some people off in the process.

As we wrap this whole thing up, I want to bring you a little bit of the magic of support groups. If you haven't heard, these groups bring together people going through similar struggles to share their stories, recent challenges, and wins, and offer authentically kind words.

Sometimes these meetings are virtual, sometimes they're in person. Some are hosted by therapists, some aren't. Regardless of the details, their goal is to make you feel less alone.

When you're dealing with mom trauma, a thing people rarely talk about, you might feel broken and alone. Support groups can change that. Hopping onto a Zoom call with twenty-five other people who get it can validate everything you've thought or felt about your mom. Sometimes it feels like the mom they're describing is *your* mom.

That normalization might be exactly what you need to overcome the stigma of not being close to your mother. Then you can get to the deeper work of accepting your mom as she is, grieving what she'll never be, setting boundaries, and living for yourself instead of your mom.

Unfortunately for me, I found this kind of support pretty late in my process. By the time I started attending group therapy, I'd finally gotten to a place where I could roll my eyes at and move on from my relationship with my mom—most of the time. But, at least for now, I still go to group. Those meetings remind me of how far I've come, and they're a source of support when my grief flares up.

Because I know how meaningful it is to find community around a thing you've been dealing with alone, I asked a few other people who can relate to share their stories. Here, they talk about the challenges they faced, the ways they cared for themselves, and how they're doing now.

Spoiler: Not everyone is completely over it. Some have been through extreme trauma, and others are still figuring out what they want their relationship with their mom to look and feel like in the future. Some are no-contact, some are low-contact, and some still talk to their moms all the time.

My intention is for you to see some part of yourself (and your mom) in these stories. Sure, maybe their mother isn't as *special* as yours, or their situation is much more extreme than what you're going through. Still, the emotional toll this dysfunctional relationship takes is what we all have in common.

I also hope you notice how these folks were able to make positive changes. What was the thing that shifted their perspective or made them feel safe putting their feelings first? I wonder if you might steal those strategies for yourself or consider what your version of that trajectory looks like. Just throwing it out there!

And while not every story has a perfect resolution, the pot of gold at the end of this shitshow is called growth. You're going to find so much of that here.

These anecdotes can serve as a helpful and hopeful reminder of how good life gets once you start down this path and find some motherfucking peace.

Britney, 35

At the worst point in our relationship, I felt like I wasn't wanted by my mom. I got the sense that she never meant to be a mother, but that she had kids and had to raise them, so that's what she did.

She did her best, but her best was always the bare minimum. When I realized that as an adult, I felt a lot of resentment about how I was parented. I felt like I was a better parent to myself than she ever was or would ever want to be. She never reached out to me or showed any interest in my life.

I wondered if my life would feel more purposeful, fulfilling, or meaningful in some way if I had been raised by someone who really wanted to get to know me and help me thrive.

My relationship with my mom has affected every part of my life: Because she's messy and disorganized, I feel uncomfortable around mess and clutter. So as an adult, I clean obsessively. Because she's also been on a diet my entire life, my relationship with food has never had boundaries. I could go on.

For a long time, I saw it as my job to try to get both of my parents to be healthier—to exercise, eat better, go to therapy. That sense of responsibility pushed me to push them, and I probably crossed some lines. That led to arguments, especially with my mom.

At a certain point, I felt like we abandoned each other. That feeling led me to deprioritize having any kind of relationship with her.

When I started therapy at thirty-two, I began inner-child work with my therapist. It was painful to revisit my childhood with my mom and reconcile how I was raised with the person I am now.

I learned that I had to parent myself and become responsible for myself at a very young age, and that made me feel resentful, abandoned, and broken. I felt guilty for even having some of these emotions. In my mind, these feelings were reserved for people who'd experienced more hardship than I had.

Therapy helped me decide to stop talking to my mom about my personal life. Without dating, work, my diet, my health, or my social plans to discuss, we were left with almost nothing to talk about, but it also helped me to stop feeling responsible for my parents' lives.

I went through the heartbreak of accepting that they could die as a result of the choices they're making, and there's nothing I can do to stop that. It was painful and freeing at the same time.

I tried to focus on giving my mom grace through this process. I tried, and still try, to accept that maybe she hadn't wanted kids, but she did her best. This kind of thinking helps me release resentment when it comes up.

We still have our struggles, though. Last year, she asked me what I wanted for my birthday, and I told her about something I'd seen on Instagram that I'd been meaning to try. We were on the phone while I was on a long drive, so she ordered it for me right then. Afterward, she made several comments about how expensive it was.

When it got delivered, I called to thank her again, and she made another comment about the price. It made me feel so weird. She used to do this when I was a kid and got a new toy, or new shoes that were over some budget that I didn't know existed.

That said, I feel at peace with our relationship now. We've actually had some growth over the past six months. We took a trip for a relative's birthday, and that was an opportunity for us to reconnect and have fun. I feel more grounded and realistic about who my mom is and isn't. I think I'm more accepting of her and of our relationship too. I can still be her daughter, but she'll never be the mom I imagined she could be, and that's fine.

If I could go back in time, I would tell myself that this is hard work, and people avoid dealing with their dysfunctional relationships for a reason. It hurts to go deep and feel pain that was sown when you were too young to remember, but getting to the other side doesn't just change your relationship with your mom, it changes your relationship with yourself. You will feel lighter, freer, and smarter. I feel a level of resolve I didn't realize I needed. ✹

Aaliyah, 43

My mother is a narcissist, and one of our biggest struggles was her inability to accept me choosing a different path from hers. She didn't raise me to be my own person—she wanted a reflection of herself. And when I refused to comply, her love turned to cruelty.

My mother's influence seeped into every part of my life. For example, she often said, "Because I love you, I can tell you the truth about yourself," before tearing me down.

That taught me to equate love with pain, to over-perform for validation, and to see volatility as normal behavior in a relationship. This bled into my career, my health, and my relationships.

When I was eighteen, I had cancer. Before my diagnosis, I could earn her approval by being thin, beautiful, and accomplished—things she could show off. But when I was ill, her concern wasn't for me. It was for the attention she got. After cancer, she no longer had use for me.

When I was twenty-eight, my mom disowned me. It felt like my world was collapsing. I had panic attacks for weeks. It took me years to come to terms with her betrayal.

After years of therapy and work, the scars linger. I've built a career and self-esteem, but relationships are still challenging. I keep attracting partners who have the same disordered patterns I grew up with. At least now I recognize it. I'm better at seeing red flags, and I've learned how to walk away sooner.

I found a psychiatrist who I saw three times a week. That year was agony, but it was also a turning point. Later, I discovered trauma-informed therapy and eye movement desensitization and reprocessing therapy—tools that helped address the emotional and psychological blocks I couldn't get over for years.

Since then, I've been in trauma-informed therapy, undoing the damage. The work isn't over, but now I have strong boundaries, financial independence, and better mental and physical health. I used to hear my mother's voice in my head all the time, but now I've built a life loud enough to drown her out.

I learned that my well-being is not negotiable. My mind, my emotions, and my body deserve care—not just the bare minimum. I learned the power and importance of a chosen family. And I've supported a lot of my friends in better understanding their dysfunctional families, which has been validating. I discovered that I am stronger, kinder, and more resilient than I realized. I refused to become bitter. That's my victory.

I've made multiple attempts to reconcile with my mother. Still, she refuses to engage in good faith and sets impossible conditions.

I'm coming to terms with the reality: Her actions reflect her brokenness, not my worth. I'm learning to accept that some people are incapable of love or accountability, and protecting myself is not only necessary but deserved. I've learned that when you grieve the mother you should've had, your life will get better. Freedom begins when you stop letting your mom define your life. ✸

Nick, 31

My relationship with my mom has felt shallow for a long time, and it's unclear why she's so emotionally unavailable. I can't tell if she genuinely doesn't care about my life or if she's emotionally immature to the point where a real conversation beyond "How's the weather?" has been impossible.

When I try to ask exploratory questions, I'm typically met with a defensive reaction. I want my mom to be curious about who I am, my friends, partners, and goals, but she isn't. It's been hard for me to set my expectations for this relationship.

After having a panic attack, I started going to therapy for intrusive thoughts. My therapist and I explored why I have a hard time talking about my feelings, a thing that likely contributed to my panic attack.

I learned that my relationship with my mom is part of the problem. It's challenged my ability to talk about in-depth, emotionally charged content, the meaningful stuff I never discussed with her.

Through therapy, I started to understand that I needed to set appropriate expectations for interactions with my mom. Part of that process included coming to terms with the fact that my mom is the way she is. She's not going to change.

The truth is, I'll probably never know why she's like that. I could assume that she doesn't care about my life or that her emotional immaturity makes her incapable of establishing deep, meaningful connections with me. I choose the latter because if I assumed she actually didn't care about me, I wouldn't want to have a relationship. I'd rather have a shallow relationship with my mom than none at all.

That said, the dynamic is forever changed. Knowing I have to lower my expectations in every conversation I have with her has helped, but it still sucks knowing this is as good as it's going to get.

If you're going through this, too, just protect yourself first. There is no relationship, whether it's with friends, partners, or family, worth sacrificing your mental health. ✹

Mariah, 39

I grew up thinking that mothers were supposed to offer unconditional love, but my relationship with my mother has always felt conditional. She said she loved me—unless she was mad at me. If I didn't meet her conditions, some of which were unspoken, her reaction was explosive. The silent treatment was a standard punishment in my house. When my brother got his first tattoo, she didn't talk to him for a year and a half.

I always felt like I was walking on eggshells around her. I know I was loved as a kid, and there were times when we were very close. She even used to say that I was her best friend. But the older I got, the more it felt like there was no pleasing her.

I think our relationship was probably fine until I got closer to adulthood and started having my own opinions, wants, and needs. She raised me to be an independent, confident person, but she expected me to act the way she would.

As an adult, I felt like everything I did disappointed her. If a relationship fell apart, she said it was because I had a wall up. If I fought with a friend, she asked what I did to them. If something was up at work, she said it was because I acted out. But when I did things I was proud of, she didn't give me any direct praise.

This relationship affected other parts of my life too. I never got apologies when she hurt my feelings, so I allowed a lot of people to treat me badly and didn't stand up for myself. Several close friendships ended as a result of my own emotional immaturity, which stemmed from my relationship with my mother.

I still haven't had a serious romantic relationship because I struggle with being vulnerable with someone new. My mom dismissed my anxiety and depression as an attitude, so I didn't get help or medications for years.

I think most people would say I'm a high-functioning person, but there's a lot of low self-worth, distrust, and fear of how I'm perceived underneath that. I've been working through it.

For a long time, I've had this sense that I owe my mom something because she's my mother. It took me a while to realize she didn't treat me badly because I'm bad. She treated me that way because of her emotional limitations. So, when I don't act how she wants, she considers it a personal affront and resorts to shaming me or giving the silent treatment.

When I reached a point where I was mentally and emotionally unwell due to my mom's expectations, I went to therapy. The therapist told me to look up "narcissistic mothers" on TikTok. When I did, it was a light bulb moment. I realized this situation wasn't unique to me. It was my mother who had a mental health problem that she was unwilling to address.

Then my therapist and I talked about boundaries. I wanted to keep my nuclear family intact, but every time I engaged with them, I left feeling bad about myself. I was always the bad guy who ended up apologizing and smoothing things over, even when my feelings had been hurt.

Thanks to years of therapy, I now realize my mother doesn't recognize that her behavior is hurtful because she thinks she is right and I'm wrong. There's no nuance. She is incapable of empathy and self-reflection, and she doesn't understand that other people have different perspectives.

I tried to work things out, with my therapist's guidance, before going no-contact. But that conversation followed the same pattern. So I decided I'd had enough.

After a holiday a couple of years ago, she sent me a passive-aggressive text saying something like "How sad and painful that you were unable to wish your family a happy holiday, wishing you love and sweetness for the year ahead. I hope you find what you're looking for."

Never mind the fact that she didn't wish me a happy holiday either! I told her if that's how she was going to speak to me, I'd rather her not speak to me at all. I haven't heard from her since.

I spent hours talking to my therapist about what kinds of behaviors are appropriate to accept and what aren't. If I'm going no-contact with my mother because of how she treated me, I'm not going to accept that treatment from anyone else.

I also got better at opening up to friends. I used to isolate myself during depressive episodes. I was afraid people would think I was being dramatic or needy. But when I started debating whether to go no-contact with my mother—a time when I was pretty depressed—I tried to be honest about what I was going through.

My therapist said again and again: "Your friends are your chosen family." I believe that now.

I'm not a bad person—I'm a human being with flaws. I guess I could say the same about my mother. But the difference is that I'm self-aware and working on addressing those flaws. She's unwilling to address her issues, and I'm not willing to put up with her as she is.

I'm in a place of acceptance right now, but there's still some anger. There's also sadness. My mother cut off her emotionally abusive parents, and it seems tragic that she's perpetuating that cycle. That said, if she is willing to take accountability and show emotional maturity, the door is open.

I feel like I've basically grieved the death of my mother. I miss the mother I wish I had, but she never existed. And even if she and I get to a place where we are in contact, it will never be the kind of mother–daughter relationship I want.

To anyone else in a similar situation: Know that you don't owe your mother anything just because she birthed you. You deserve to be in relationships where both people are doing the work to keep it healthy. If your relationship with your mother is having a negative effect on the rest of your life, talk to a professional. Surround yourself with people who support you. And if you have to make the hard decision to go no-contact, that's OK. You're not alone. ✹

ACKNOWLEDGMENTS

First, thank you to my therapist for asking me years ago, "What do you want to do with all of this?" Rachel, it's done! Your insights, gold stars, and gentle nudges are worth a lifetime of co-pays. I am endlessly grateful for the work you do.

The other reason this book exists is my unstoppable agent, Jill Marsal. Thank you for having my back and chilling me out in the thick of this process. I am blessed to have you in my corner.

To my editors, Leah Wilson and Victoria Carmody, thank you for your smart notes, genius edits, and all the :) in the comments. You two get me, and you'll never know just how much I appreciate that! Another shout-out to Clara Tamez, who helped this book through the final stages of the process!

Additional gratitude to the entire team at BenBella, especially Sarah Avinger, Kim Broderick, Heather Butterfield, Jennifer Canzoneri, Morgan Carr, James Fraleigh, Madeline Grigg, Alicia Kania, Adrienne Lang, Lindsay Marshall, Rachel Phares, and Susan Welte.

To the incomparable experts who graciously lent me their time and expertise—Minaa B., Dr. Claudia Brumbaugh, Whitney Goodman, Dr. Kathryn Humphreys, Dr. Robert A. Neimeyer, Vienna Pharaon, and

Dr. Jenny Tzu-Mei Wang—I cannot thank you all enough. Working on this project with you helped me heal, and I know it will do the same for countless others. You're all the damn best. Seriously.

A reporter is nothing without backup (dumb journalism pun intended). Lauren Dzubow and Sal Tamarkin, thank you for your diligent review of my drafts. I sleep better at night because of the work you two did here and continue to do in the world. Fact checkers fucking rule!

To team Wondermind (past, present, and future), thank you for your bottomless support and encouragement. An extra special shout out to: Mandy Teefey, Selena Gomez, Daniella Pierson, Bhavik Trevidi, Jessica Schiffer, Jordan Fink, Claudia Lewis, Lauren Pyo, Johnathan Glucksman, and Emma Wright.

My chosen family and cheering squad believed in me more than I believed in myself. Thank you for the milestone celebrations and antidepressant recommendations. I wouldn't have pursued either without you all: Tatiana Imamura-Hogan, Rachel Torgerson, Christina Bellin, Allison Berry, Jessica Goodman, Annie Davalle Durling, Dani Martinson, Max Rakhlenko, Joe Navarre, Preston Kemp, Steph Rickards, Nikki Espina, Chris Godburn, Jenny Cook, James Rignall, Meghan DiSanto, Jenni Ryan, Erika Ratz, Kayla Logan, Elly Corrigan, Angela Wiebel, and Samantha Vlado.

Sascha de Gersdorff, Meredith Bryan, Rosa Heyman, Jess Giles, and Casey Gueren are the mentors I'm now lucky enough to call friends. Thank you all for helping me find my voice as a writer and editor. You're the reason this book sounds so unhinged. (CG, I would be lost without you!)

To Nana, love you more!

Thank you to my brother Chad. I've rewritten this sentence like eight times now, and no version was good enough. So, just know that I love you, bruh. To my mom and dad, thank you for being brave! I know this wasn't easy. Still, neither of you doubted me for a second. I hope I made you proud. Love you both!

Sean Meyer, I can barely remember the worst parts of this process, but I'll never forget the ways you helped me through. When we crack the good champagne, I'll be raising a glass to you. Love you, boo.

ABOUT THE AUTHOR

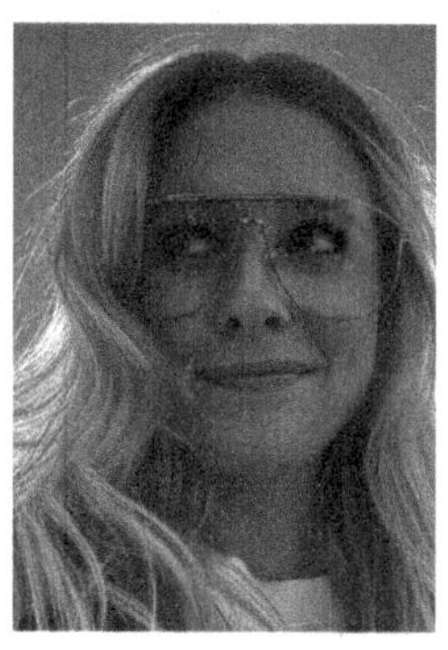

Ashley Oerman is a reporter, writer, and editor with a focus on health, wellness, and lifestyle content at brands like *Cosmopolitan*, where she was the brand's lifestyle director. During her nearly five years at *Cosmopolitan*, Ashley's work was nominated for a National Magazine Award for personal service. She's also held editorial positions at *Women's Health* magazine and *Parents*.

Now, as the deputy editor at Wondermind, a mental health-centered media company founded by Selena Gomez and Mandy Teefey, she edits and writes deeply helpful, easy-to-understand mental health content and develops the brand's editorial strategy. Since 2012, her work has reached millions of eyes across the US and internationally.